ICRU REPORT 54

Medical Imaging—The Assessment of Image Quality

Issued: 8 April 1996

INTERNATIONAL COMMISSION ON RADIATION
UNITS AND MEASUREMENTS
7910 WOODMONT AVENUE
BETHESDA, MARYLAND 20814
U.S.A.

THE INTERNATIONAL COMMISSION
ON RADIATION UNITS AND MEASUREMENTS

INDIVIDUALS PARTICIPATING IN THE PREPARATION OF THIS REPORT

The Commission wishes to express its appreciation to the individuals involved in the preparation of this Report for the time and effort which they devoted to this task and to express its appreciation to the organizations with which they are affiliated.

(For detailed information of the availability of this and other ICRU Reports, see page 82.)

Preface

Scope of ICRU Activities

The International Commission on Radiation Units and Measurements (ICRU), since its inception in 1925, has had as its principal objective the development of internationally acceptable recommendations regarding:

1. Quantities and units of radiation and radioactivity,
2. Procedures suitable for the measurement and application of these quantities in clinical radiology and radiobiology and
3. Physical data needed in the application of these procedures, the use of which tends to assure uniformity in reporting.

The Commission also considers and makes similar types of recommendations for the radiation protection field. In this connection, its work is carried out in close cooperation with the International Commission on Radiological Protection (ICRP).

Policy

The ICRU endeavors to collect and evaluate the latest data and information pertinent to the problems of radiation measurement and dosimetry and to recommend the most acceptable values and techniques for current use.

The Commission's recommendations are kept under continual review in order to keep abreast of the rapidly expanding uses of radiation.

The ICRU feels that it is the responsibility of national organizations to introduce their own detailed technical procedures for the development and maintenance of standards. However, it urges that all countries adhere as closely as possible to the internationally recommended basic concepts of radiation quantities and units.

The Commission feels that its responsibility lies in developing a system of quantities and units having the widest possible range of applicability. Situations may arise from time to time when an expedient solution of a current problem may seem advisable. Generally speaking, however, the Commission feels that action based on expediency is inadvisable from a long-term viewpoint; it endeavors to base its decision on the long-range advantages to be expected.

The ICRU invites and welcomes constructive comments and suggestions regarding its recommendations and reports. These may be transmitted to the Chairman.

Current Program

The Commission has divided its field of interest into 12 technical areas and has assigned one or more members of the Commission the responsibility for identification of potential topics for new ICRU activities in each area. Each area is reviewed periodically by its sponsors. Recommendations for new reports are then reviewed by the Commission and a priority assigned. The technical areas are:

Radiation Therapy
Diagnostic Radiology
Nuclear Medicine
Radiobiology
Radioactivity
Radiation Physics— X Rays, Gamma Rays and Electrons
Radiation Physics— Neutrons and Heavy Particles
Radiation Protection
Radiation Chemistry
Critical Data
Theoretical Aspects
Quantities and Units

The actual preparation of ICRU reports is carried out by ICRU report committees. One or more Commission members serve as sponsors to each committee and provide close liaison with the Commission. The currently active report committees are:

Absorbed Dose Standards for Photon Irradiation and Their Dissemination
Beta-Ray Dosimetry for Radiation Protection
Clinical Dosimetry for Neutrons (Specification of Beam Quality)
Determination of Body Burdens for Radionuclides
Dose Specification for Reporting Interstitial Therapy
Dosimetric Procedures in Diagnostic Radiology
Fundamental Quantities and Units
Mammography — Assessment of Image Quality
Medical Application of Beta Rays
Nuclear Data
Prescribing, Recording and Reporting Electron Beam Therapy
Proton Therapy
ROC Analysis
Radiobiology Specification of Beam Quality and Specification of Therapy Parameters
Relationship between Quantities for Radiological Protection against External Radiation (Joint ICRP-ICRU Task Group)
Requirements for Radioecological Sampling
Secondary Electron Spectra Resulting from Charged Particle Interactions
Statistical Aspects of Environmental Sampling
Stopping Power for Heavy Ions
Tissue Substitutes, Characteristics of Biological Tissue and Phantoms for Ultrasound

ICRU's Relationships with Other Organizations

In addition to its close relationship with the ICRP, the ICRU has developed relationships with other organizations interested in the problems of radiation quantities, units and measurements. Since 1955, the ICRU has had an official relationship with the World Health Organization (WHO), whereby the ICRU is looked to for primary guidance in matters of radiation units and measurements and, in turn, the WHO assists in the world-wide dissemination of the Commission's recommendations. In 1960, the ICRU entered into consultative status with the International Atomic Energy Agency. The Commission has a formal relationship with the United Nations Scientific Committee on the Effects of Atomic Radiation (UNSCEAR), whereby ICRU observers are invited to attend UNSCEAR meetings. The Commission and the International Organization for Standardization (ISO) informally exchange notifications of meetings, and the ICRU is formally designated for liaison with two of the ISO technical committees. The ICRU also corresponds and exchanges final reports with the following organizations:

> Bureau International de Métrologie Légale
> Bureau International des Poids et Mesures
> Commission of the European Communities
> Council for International Organizations of Medical Sciences
> Food and Agriculture Organization of the United Nations
> International Council of Scientific Unions
> International Electrotechnical Commission
> International Labor Office
> International Organization for Medical Physics
> International Radiation Protection Association
> International Union of Pure and Applied Physics
> United Nations Educational, Scientific and Cultural Organization

The Commission has found its relationship with all of these organizations fruitful and of substantial benefit to the ICRU program. Relations with these other international bodies do not affect the basic affiliation of the ICRU with the International Society of Radiology.

Operating Funds

In the early days of its existence, the ICRU operated essentially on a voluntary basis, with the travel and operating costs being borne by the parent organization of the participants. (Only token assistance was originally available from the International Society of Radiology.) Recognizing the impractibility of continuing this mode of operation on an indefinite basis, operating funds were sought from various sources.

During the last 10 years, financial support has been received from the following organizations:

> American Society for Therapeutic Radiology and Oncology
> Atomic Energy Control Board
> Bayer AG
> Central Electricity Generating Board
> Commissariat à l'Énergie Atomique
> Commission of the European Communities
> Dutch Society for Radiodiagnostics
> Eastman Kodak Company
> Ebara Corporation
> Électricité de France
> Fuji Medical Systems
> General Electric Company
> Hitachi, Ltd.
> International Atomic Energy Agency
> International Radiation Protection Association
> International Society of Radiology
> Italian Radiological Association
> Japan Industries Association of Radiation Apparatus
> Konica Corporation
> National Cancer Institute of the U.S. Department of Health and Human Services
> National Electrical Manufacturers Association
> Philips Medical Systems, Incorporated
> Radiation Research Society
> Scanditronix AB
> Siemens Aktiengesellschaft
> Sumitomo Heavy Industries, Ltd.
> Theratronics
> Toshiba Corporation
> University Hospital Lund, Sweden
> World Health Organization

In addition to the direct monetary support provided by these organizations, many organizations provide indirect support for the Commission's program. This support is provided in many forms, including, among others, subsidies for (1) the time of individuals participating in ICRU activities, (2) travel costs involved in ICRU meetings and (3) meeting facilities and services.

In recognition of the fact that its work is made possible by the generous support provided by all of the organizations supporting its program, the Commission expresses its deep appreciation.

André Allisy
Chairman, ICRU

Sèvres, France
15 March 1996

Contents

Executive Summary

There have been dramatic improvements in medical imaging capability over the past two decades, particularly due to the utilization of digital technology. One consequence is the challenge that this has posed to the process of assessing the performance of imaging systems, especially the measurement of the comparative efficacy of various modalities. This Report proposes a framework, based on statistical decision theory, within which imaging system performance may be measured, optimized and compared.

Imaging system assessment depends on the task for which the system is intended and can, therefore, be cast in terms of task performance. This performance can be measured in two stages. First, task performance can be measured in terms of how well an ideal or Bayesian decision maker would perform the task using only the acquired data, *i.e.*, before it is presented as an image to a human observer. This can be done for certain well-defined imaging tasks, and leads to a description of the quality of the acquired data in terms of an ideal observer signal-to-noise ratio.

The second stage involves measurement of the performance of the task by observers using displayed data. In this case, the assessment is made in terms of a receiver operating characteristic (ROC) curve and the quality of the displayed data can be specified in terms of a signal-to-noise ratio.

The two stages of performance assessment are complementary and their related roles are explored in this Report. The analysis of the acquired data has the advantage of allowing one to investigate the effect on performance of altering various parameters of the imaging system. In certain circumstances, this approach may permit calculation of the best achievable signal-to-noise ratio, but at present it does not necessarily predict the behavior of the human observer. This approach also requires laboratory measurements of system parameters such as modulation transfer function and noise power or Wiener spectrum and these might require special resources. The ROC curve approach provides a thorough assessment of the quality of the displayed data that takes the observer's behavior into account, but it may be demanding of time and resources. Thus, it is proposed that the analysis based on the acquired data may provide not only an assessment of the potential performance of the imaging system, but also guidance as to those imaging conditions under which it would be most profitable to perform the ROC analysis.

Finally, the proposed framework links the purely objective measures of device performance to the subjective assessment of image quality and, further, offers the potential for moving to higher levels of efficacy analysis involving cost-benefit analysis of clinical data.

List of Symbols and Abbreviations

A_Z	area under the ROC curve
$\mathbf{C}$	covariance
d', d_a	effective signal-to-noise ratio
$\mathbf{f}$	object data
FPF	false positive fraction
$\mathbf{g}$	image data
$\mathbf{H}$	system transfer function
H_K	kth hypothesis
K	large-area transfer factor
L	likelihood ratio
L_C	likelihood ratio threshold
LSF	line spread function
MAFC	multi-alternative forced choice
MAP	maximum *a posteriori* (estimator)
MSE	mean squared error
MTF	modulation transfer function
NEQ	noise equivalent quanta
NPS	noise power spectrum
NPWMF	nonprewhitening matched filter
OTF	optical transfer function
PSF	point spread function
PWMF	prewhitening matched filter
ROC	receiver operating characteristic (curve)
SNR	signal-to-noise ratio
TPF	true positive fraction
W	Wiener spectrum
2AFC	two alternative forced choice
γ	film gamma
κ	incremental-signal transfer factor
ν	spatial frequency

Medical Imaging—The Assessment of Image Quality

1. General Introduction

1.1 Preamble

During the past two decades, the field of medical imaging has achieved dramatic improvements in imaging system capability with accompanying increases in system complexity. Much of this progress has been fueled by advances in computing technology and the widespread adoption of digital techniques for data acquisition, processing and display. Although every branch of medical imaging has been significantly affected, the most striking examples of this revolution are x-ray computed tomography and magnetic resonance imaging. An overview of these and other major medical diagnostic imaging modalities is given in Appendix A.

The pace of change in this field has presented an enormous challenge to the process of technology assessment. Questions of comparative efficacy between modalities and system optimization within each modality require timely resolution, but it is frequently unclear as how best to address them. Clinical trials are an obvious way to test the effectiveness of new techniques. Such studies are both expensive and time consuming, however, and the technologies they seek to monitor present moving targets; by the time the studies have been completed, the technologies have taken evolutionary steps forward. Alternatives to clinical trials have been offered by laboratory investigators in the form of physical measurements, such as spatial resolution and noise level, on imaging systems or components, but these approaches are challenged by the issue of how to relate these measures to the clinical performance of the systems.

Fortunately, a consensus on quantitative measurement methodology for assessing diagnostic imaging technologies has been gradually emerging. It has grown out of the recognition of common features among imaging modalities that allows their limitations to be understood within the framework of statistical decision analysis.

1.2 The Problem of Defining the Quality of the Image

A medical image is a representation of the distribution of some property of the human body which shows the structure and/or function of organs and tissues under investigation. The diversity of possible structures and functions relevant to clinical diagnosis places a wide variety of requirements on any imaging system. For example, the detection of microcalcifications in mammography requires that very fine detail be preserved, so high contrast and high spatial resolution are needed. On the other hand, the identification of hemorrhage in x-ray computed tomography (CT) of the head requires sensitivity to small contrast differences, but is frequently not demanding of fine spatial resolution. Thus, any general definition of image quality must address the effectiveness with which the image can be used for its intended task.

Imaging systems are often described in terms of physical quantities that characterize various aspects of their performance. These include measures of contrast in the image between different tissues [or tissue substitutes (ICRU,1988)], the detailed nature of system spatial resolution (ICRU,1986) and the quantity and character of the image noise. A task-based measure of system performance will depend on these physical parameters, as well as on the detailed nature of the diagnostic task, including the complexities arising from the variability and overlap of tissues and anatomical structures, and the degree to which information provided by the imaging system is perceived by the clinician.

The complexity of the diagnostic task and the physical design of the imaging system impose limitations on the fundamental quality of the detected image data. Even so, the ability of the human observer to utilize a displayed version of the data can frequently be the limiting factor affecting diagnostic outcome. Although, in principle, digital image display capability should lead to optimal extraction of detected information by the reader, in practice it can just as well impede this process. For example, it is not too difficult to manipulate a displayed image, by contrast enhancement and gray-level thresholding, in such a way that relevant clinical details are no longer perceptible in the image. Thus, it cannot always be assumed that the quality of the displayed image reflects the quality of the data acquired by the imaging device. For this reason the imaging process is conceived of as taking place in two stages: data is first detected or captured from a stream of radiation; the detected image is then processed and displayed. This dichotomy, which was subtle to appreciate before the computer came to play a crucial role in imaging systems, is now quite obvious in the case of digital systems. Each stage of the imaging system can be evaluated by the measurement or calculation of a given observer's ability to perform a particular task. This Report will offer a methodology for the separate assessment of these two stages in the imaging process.

1.3 The Decision-Making Paradigm

A straightforward paradigm from the theory of statistical decision making is used as the foundation for much of this Report. This paradigm provides the framework for quantitative, task-based image assessment of both the detection stage and display stage of an imaging system. To assess an imaging system in this manner a task must first be specified, and then the ability of some observer (decision maker), such as a radiologist, to perform the task using the image data, either as detected or as finally displayed by the system, must be determined.

The tasks considered in this Report can be categorized as classification and estimation. Classification involves assigning an image to one of a limited number of possible groups or classes. In its simplest form, classification becomes the task of detection, the classification being into one of two classes: either the image shows a deviation from the normal structure or it is normal. Thus, detection is the clinical problem of identifying that, e.g., there is a metastasis present in a radionuclide bone scan or a lung nodule in a chest radiograph. On the other hand, estimation involves measuring the value of some (continuously variable) parameter calculable from information in the image, e.g., the degree of renal stenosis demonstrated in a renal arteriogram. The problem of estimation will be

further considered in Section 3.8 and Appendix H, but as there is currently no clear agreement on how it should be evaluated, only classification will be dealt with in detail in this Report.

For a binary diagnostic decision, e.g., classification of an image as either normal or abnormal, the statistical decision theory approach assumes that an observer determines a decision variable that is used to classify each image. For example, blood sugar content or serum cholesterol level are simple decision variables used in laboratory diagnostic testing, providing the basis for decisions on the presence or absence of abnormal conditions. The much more complex judgements by a radiologist of the amount of unusual darkening, lightening or texture in a region in a radiograph represent decision variables in medical imaging.

The decision paradigm presupposes the existence of an actually normal and an actually abnormal population, both of which generate a spread (or distribution) of decision variable outcomes, or readings, as shown in Figure 1.1. Thus, as the task is to classify an image as either normal or abnormal, image quality is determined by the degree of overlap of these two populations. As the readings for the two populations commonly overlap, as shown in the figure, a statistical approach is required to assess image quality. Image quality may not be judged adequately on the basis of a single image; information derived from a set of images is required to determine the usefulness of the imaging system in separating the underlying populations.

To classify an image, the observer or decision maker adopts some value of the decision variable as a threshold; readings on one side of this threshold are reported as abnormal, those on the other side as normal. This threshold will lead to a particular

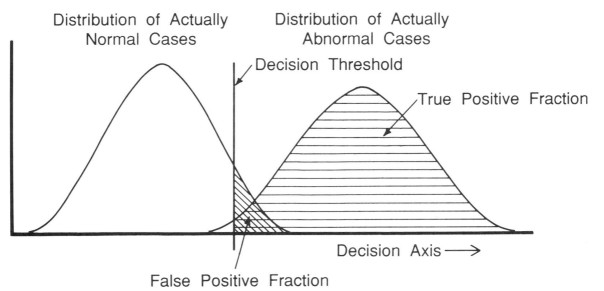

Fig. 1.1. The statistical decision theory paradigm.

proportion of actually abnormal images being correctly reported as abnormal — the true positive fraction (TPF) (sensitivity) — and a certain proportion of actually normal images being incorrectly classified as abnormal — the false positive fraction (FPF) (one minus specificity). As the decision threshold is varied, the TPFs and FPFs will also change. The curve showing the TPF as a function of the FPF is known as the receiver operating characteristic (ROC) curve. This curve translates the overlap of the two populations into a quantitative measure of image quality.

The detailed motivation and practical implementation of the ROC methodology is the subject of Section 4. Several summary measures of performance derived from the ROC curve are presented there. One of these, d_a, has the general form of a signal to noise ratio (SNR) for the detection of an abnormality (or discrimination between types of abnormalities). It expresses the separation of the two distributions, for the normal and abnormal populations (the signal), in units of the noise defined as the average spread (root-mean-square standard deviation) of the two populations. This SNR is potentially a very useful concept for providing a summary measure of image quality.

There are several factors contributing to the spread of the decision variables and it is, in principle, possible to separate their contribution to an overall signal-to-noise ratio. The major contributions to the spread are shown in Figure 1.2: the random fluctuations that naturally occur in the process of data acquisition (*e.g.*, photon noise); biological variations both within the patient and among the patients in the population; artifacts due to the inadequacy of the data that remain during the process of image formation; and intra- and inter-observer variability. Estimates of the separate contributions of these factors to overall imaging performance may be achieved by defining several categories of decision makers that

have access to the image information at different stages of the imaging process.

1.4 Decision Makers

Decision variable distributions depend upon the type of observer, or decision maker, who formulates them and the stage of the imaging system at which they are applied. The imaging process is conceived as taking place in two stages: data are first detected or captured from a stream of radiation; the detected image is then processed and displayed. To evaluate the quality of the detection stage, where the image may not be a recognizable picture of the human body [as in CT and magnetic resonance imaging (MRI)], certain mathematical model observers are defined and the system is assessed on the ability of these observers to perform specific tasks using the raw data. The display stage is evaluated with human observers.

1.4.1 The Ideal Decision Maker

The detection stage of the imaging process can be assessed by invoking the ideal observer from Bayesian decision theory who forms an optimal decision function (see Appendix C) and makes a decision based on the detected image data. This decision maker yields the best possible discrimination between data classes and sometimes can be implemented by techniques involving various matched filters derived from communications theory. This is discussed further in Section 3.

The assessment of ideal-observer performance generally addresses the spread in the two populations due to the random variations — so-called stochastic noise — that occur in the process of image detection. This performance is usually calculated for simple idealized phantoms (Section 4.4). The evaluation

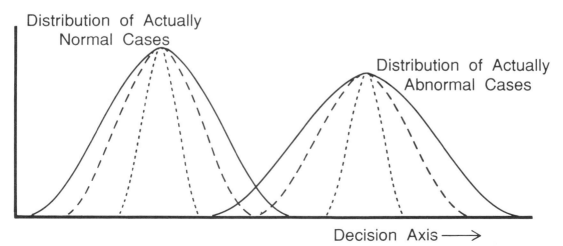

Fig. 1.2. The various factors contributing to the spread of the decision variables: spread from random noise fluctuations (- - - -), that from noise and biological variability (– – – –), that from noise, biological variability, artifacts and observer variability (——).

requires measurements of the intrinsic contrast of the feature, such as a lesion, being detected (*i.e.*, the signal), the contrast transfer function of the imaging system, and the noise power spectrum (NPS) at a given imaging condition. These fundamental measurements and their normalization for portability between laboratories will be described in Section 3.2. These measurements are the ingredients required to calculate the SNR that determines the intrinsic detectability of a lesion in a simple phantom, the so-called ideal observer signal-to-noise ratio.

1.4.2 Quasi-Ideal Observers

While the strength of the ideal observer model is that it indicates the best possible performance, its application is usually limited to simple phantoms and decision tasks because of the difficulty of specifying it for more complicated tasks. While sacrificing the ideal nature of the analysis it is possible to modify this observer to give model decision makers which are applicable to a wider range of tasks and which may, in principle, more closely approximate the performance of human observers. Several such models are reviewed in Section 3.5. A method is also presented for directly measuring the SNRs of these observers without requiring the full set of physical measurements needed to calculate the ideal-observer performance. These observers are based on matched filters and various discriminant functions (*e.g.*, Hotelling/ Fisher). They can be used to assess the contributions to the separation of image classes from the combination of random or stochastic noise and the deterministic artifacts that arise in the detection and formation of images. Work is also presented to show how well these models correlate with the performance of a human observer.

1.4.3 Human Observers

While model observers are useful for providing a rapid assessment of performance, they are still limited to relatively simple tasks. To incorporate the complete realm of clinical complexity it is necessary to present images to a human observer and analyze performance by psychophysical techniques. The most rigorous of these, the only one allowing performance to be separated from the observer's bias, is the application of the ROC methodology. This is described in detail in Section 4. In such studies, the observer is asked to perform some visual task, and, through training, develops a decision strategy for doing so. An important aspect of psychophysical studies of image quality is that they can use real clinical images of patients, incorporating the naturally occurring biological variability to arrive at a realistic task.

1.5 Image Quality and the Diagnostic Process

Image assessment is defined here in terms of the performance of well-defined signal detection tasks. Physical performance assessment is often specified in terms of the detection or discrimination of simulated lesions while clinical performance assessment is specified in terms of the detection or discrimination of clinical lesions or other disease states. These tasks are only part of the larger clinical task, or process, that involves the management of the patient and the determination of the patient outcome and its effect on society. These issues come under the broader heading referred to as efficacy.

Fryback and Thornbury (1991) have proposed a six-level model of efficacy and this is summarized in Table 1.1. The two lowest levels are the concern of this Report, namely technical efficacy (*i.e.*, physical image performance assessment) and diagnostic accuracy (*i.e.*, clinical image performance assessment). A major purpose of this Report is to present consensus methodology so that these levels of efficacy may be characterized quantitatively. It is to be expected, furthermore, that the quantification at the first level will serve as a specification of the state of technology that can be used to label or normalize studies at the second level, and ultimately to understand their ranking of imaging systems. Similarly, quantification at both of these lower levels can serve to label or normalize studies at higher levels and contribute toward the understanding of their results. Work at all of these levels, then, represents major efforts towards a quantitative science of medical decision making.

1.6 Outline of the Report

The intention of this Report is to present a framework within which the diagnostic quality of images produced by a variety of clinical imaging devices can be evaluated. It is not proposed to deal with the detail of how this framework can be applied to each modality; although examples are given in Appendix D, this task will be tackled in subsequent reports.

TABLE 1.1—*Six-tier model of efficacy*

Level	Typical Output Measures
Technical efficacy	MTF; Gray scale steps
Diagnostic accuracy efficacy	Sensitivity, specificity, ROC curve analysis
Diagnostic thinking efficacy	Entropy change; Change in clinician's diagnostic probability
Therapeutic efficacy	Percentage of times therapy changed
Patient outcome efficacy	Change in quality adjusted life years
Societal efficacy	Summed quality adjusted years; Positive change in national product

It is suggested that, using the paradigm of statistical decision theory, the quality can be measured for both the displayed image, as viewed by the human observer, and for the acquired data, that is, the image data prior to display. In both cases, a SNR may be calculated which, for the acquired data, may, in certain circumstances, be the optimum or maximum value achievable. It will be suggested that this general approach provides comprehensive measures of image quality.

For the benefit of the reader who is not conversant with medical imaging, an introduction to the basic principles of commonly used medical imaging techniques is given in Appendix A together with comments on the applicability of the proposed process for measuring quality. Also, in Appendix B, there is a general discussion of the various types of image degradation.

The currently used measures of image quality will be reviewed in Section 2 and the approaches to be recommended in this Report will be given in Sections 3 and 4.

Section 3 describes how the performance of the imaging device may be assessed by measuring the SNR achieved when an ideal or quasi-ideal observer analyzes the acquired data. The mathematical concepts underlying this ideal or Bayesian observer are given in Sections 3.2 and 3.3, and presented more rigorously in Appendix C. Section 3.4 outlines the potential value of the quantity noise equivalent quanta (NEQ) for describing imaging system performance.

In Section 3.5, two non-ideal observer models are outlined which may be useful in circumstances where the ideal observer model is not readily calculable, or where a model is required which approximates more closely to human performance. These concepts are developed in mathematical detail in appendices E, F and G. Finally, in Section 3.8 and Appendix H, a brief consideration is given to the problem of estimation.

Section 4 deals with the assessment of the displayed image by the human observer. Section 4.2.2 describes how ROC curves are generated and Section 4.2.3 defines various indices of performance which can be derived from them. A discussion of different types of test patterns for visual assessment is given in Section 4.4.

General guidance on the practical implementation of these techniques, in a form which can be adopted by the potential user, is given in Section 5.

The concluding section emphasizes how the techniques may be developed so as to apply to more sophisticated problems of clinical diagnosis.

An alphabetic glossary is provided in Appendix I.

The point has been made that a measure of image quality is meaningful only when related to a particular task. It is the intention of this Report to suggest a framework within which the diagnostic quality of images produced by a variety of clinical imaging devices can be evaluated; any proposals for judging quality must fit into the wider process of clinical efficacy assessment (Fryback and Thornbury, 1991; Thornbury, 1994).

2. Present Approaches to Measuring Image Quality Parameters

2.1 Introduction

A variety of techniques for measuring the performance of imaging systems has evolved. In general, these involve presenting a known input to the imaging system and using the resulting image(s) to assess performance. This assessment may be done subjectively or using any of a wide range of degrees of objectivity. It may involve the participation of human observers or use mathematical models. It may apply to the entire imaging system or only to a part of it.

Clearly, objective measures of image quality are desirable in order to characterize the performance of an imaging system and not simply that of a particular set of observers. On the other hand, even relatively simple interpretation tasks are difficult to model realistically, so it may prove problematical to extrapolate from objective measures of quality to performance in the clinical situation. Subjective methods have the advantage that clinical utility can be assessed more directly, but it is not easy to achieve controlled test conditions and, as a consequence, results may be difficult to interpret. Since, as was noted in the previous section, image quality must relate to a clearly defined image interpretation task, the ability to relate the performance measurement to a task must be a fundamental criterion against which quality assessment methodologies should be judged.

The purpose of this Section is to describe some of the techniques commonly used for the assessment of the performance of imaging systems. These range from simple, subjective ones to the highly sophisticated methods outlined in detail in the following two sections. Deficiencies of the simple methods are noted and an indication of the rationale underlying those to be recommended is given.

2.2 Physical Image Assessment Methods

Physical image assessment is accomplished by measuring certain physical parameters and combining them according to the requirements of a particular imaging task. This may involve using one or more models of observers to calculate performance, such as the ideal Bayesian observer and other (quasi-ideal) observers.

2.2.1 Physical Parameters

There are three kinds of physical parameters which are fundamental to imaging system specification. These are:

1. Large-scale (macro) system transfer function (characteristic curve) which measures the relationship between system input, *e.g.*, exposure quanta, and the output image, *e.g.*, optical density
2. Spatial resolution properties
3. Noise properties

These parameters are required for any serious determination of system performance, but they are largely task independent and, thus, by themselves, do not provide any definitive way of rating or ranking systems. They do, however, serve as the basic means of system specification and as the building blocks for more complete performance appraisal. Note, however, that these tools do not cover image dependent artifacts, such as aliasing due to undersampling. Some of these problems are considered in Section 3.

The large-scale transfer function is a prerequisite for quantitative performance analysis since it provides the relationship between values in the object and those measured in the output image. For many systems this is not a simple linear relationship, but non-linear, such as logarithmic.

Systematic image degradation due to spatial resolution properties can be characterized effectively by observing the response of a system to known, simple objects. In principle, such information can be used to predict the response to more complex objects. The point spread function (PSF), line spread function (LSF) and edge spread function (ESF) are the responses of a system to point, line and step-edge objects, respectively. In each case, a highly localized feature will generally produce a blurred image which defines the degree of spatial correlation. The modulation transfer function (MTF) of a system is defined as its response to a sinusoidal input; it specifies the relative amplitude of the output signal as a function of the spatial frequency of the sinusoid. In general, the response will decrease as the frequency increases. The MTF can be derived simply by computing the two-dimensional Fourier transform of the PSF or, more commonly, by the one-dimensional transform of the line spread function (Metz and Doi, 1979). Issues that must be addressed in calculating and interpreting the transfer functions of digital imaging systems are discussed in Giger and Doi (1984) and Metz (1985).

The introduction of noise into an imaging process means that the system is no longer deterministic and that its performance must be analyzed using statistical methods. The simplest measure of output noise is given by the variance of the intensity over the image of a uniform object. This description is, however, incomplete because it does not specify the spatial correlation of the noise. This is an important omission since interactions between the spatial structure of the noise, the structure of the signal and the imaging blur are major causes of irreversible image degradation. The spatial correlation of noise can be fully characterized for most important cases by its Wiener spectrum which measures the noise power as a function of spatial frequency (Giger *et al.*, 1984). The Wiener spectrum is also the Fourier transform of the noise autocorrelation function (see Section 3.2.3).

2.2.2 Difference Metrics

The most direct method of evaluating image quality, in the sense of fidelity to the original object, is to determine the mean squared error (MSE). This involves computing the average, over the image format, of the square of the difference between the output image of the system and the image that a perfect system would have provided of the same object. This represents the degree of difference between the images from the actual and ideal systems. Mean squared error (which is closely related to the cross-correlation of the two images) and other point difference metrics are superficially attractive, but have limited practical value because they fail to differentiate between quite different forms of degradation. For example, many small differences can give the same value of MSE as one large difference, and a simple uniform contrast or position off-set would yield a large value of MSE, but be completely irrelevant to performance on most imaging tasks. This figure of merit is, however, useful for tasks involving estimation.

2.2.3 Statistical Decision Theory

Modern image evaluation methodology has developed from concepts based on statistical decision theory. These concepts arose naturally during the evolution of modern communications engineering, where message transmission and reception with low probability of error is the desired goal. Military and commercial applications abound, and major developments were made in applications to diagnostic medicine and psychology. Statistical decision theory, and the related field of information theory, find a natural application in the assessment of the performance of imaging systems. These fields address the problem of making the best possible choice among several alternatives when given a certain amount of information. Thus, specifying a task and specifying the capabilities of the observer using the imaging system leads naturally to the question of how the system performs in providing the observer with the information it can use to accomplish the task.

Methods of system assessment based on information theory and those based on statistical decision theory converge to the measures of SNR that are discussed in Section 3. A critical component of this approach is the type of decision maker, or observer

model, used and a few general comments concerning this are given below.

2.2.3.1 Ideal Observer Formalism. The ideal Bayesian observer is one who is able to use all the information available in carrying out the imaging task. The ideal observer can correctly account for correlations in the noise and is unaffected by any reversible (information conserving) image processing. It does as well as any observer possibly can do (in a minimum cost or error sense), and its performance can be measured at any stage in the imaging system as a measure of the task-related information transmitted by the system up through that stage.

2.2.3.2 Other Observers. For complicated tasks, calculation of the ideal observer performance measure may not be tractable, and other, more easily calculable, models may be required. In addition, the human observer is not ideal, in particular, lacking the ability to account effectively for (or prewhiten) correlations in image noise. For these reasons, various model observers, with characteristics more closely tuned to those of the human observer, are frequently used to infer human performance. Two such observers, the Hotelling observer and the NPWMF, are discussed in Section 3 and Appendices E and F.

2.3 Psychophysical Approaches

Psychophysical approaches to the evaluation of imaging system performance measure the performance of real observers, often on real clinical tasks.

2.3.1 Subjective Assessment of Image Quality

"Subjective" refers to individual human judgement, so in a strict sense all methods employing human observers are subjective. Techniques have been developed, however, to distill quantitative, objective results from human observer studies; the present Section discusses those techniques in which observer preference is the primary element.

Subjective judgement is subject to sources of bias ranging from preference for the aesthetically pleasing to prejudice against the unfamiliar, and thus potentially provides the least reliable assessment of image quality. On the other hand, it may be fast, easy to do and, at least for experienced observers, provide an early indication of the strengths and weaknesses of an imaging system. It is clearly of potential value in two circumstances. Firstly, when no objective method is available, usually because the technology of a new imaging modality or technique is evolving too rapidly to allow a statistically useful sample of images to be collected under controlled conditions. Secondly, it may provide an insight into factors influencing image quality which may be missed by approaches using too rigidly defined study protocols.

One potentially useful approach in such situations involves subjective comparisons of image quality in which the observer's attention is focused systematically upon specific normal or pathological anatomical features in similar views of a particular patient imaged with two modalities (Vucich, 1979). After attending to each feature, the observer is required to report the relative fidelity with which it is demonstrated by the two modalities, using a five- or seven-point rating scale, for example. Although results obtained in this way are inevitably subject to bias and variations in different observers' use of the scale on which impressions are reported, the use of a common patient sample and the act of focusing attention on specific image features may help to guard against gross violations of objectivity.

A second technique involves the observer ranking versions of the same image, differing according to some imaging parameter, using a specific criterion such as image sharpness. Comparison of the rank order produced for many different images allows one to test for particular preferences for images displayed in one certain way. This has, e.g., been applied to the study of the effect of image pixel size on image quality, the ranking criteria being observer preference (Sharp et al., 1982). The development of techniques for "multidimensional scaling" (MDS) may also be of benefit to these rank-order type studies. Given rank ordering of image preference or similarity judgements, MDS techniques determine the number of relevant dimensions that yield the subjective determination of image preference or similarity (Kruskal and Wish, 1978).

2.3.2 Method of Constant Stimulus

Historically, many experiments in the field of psychophysics have used the "method of constant stimulus," in which a sensory signal with constant characteristics is presented to an observer on multiple occasions. After each trial, the observer is required to report whether the signal, which was, in fact, always present, had been "detected." The level of performance achieved by the observer is represented by the fraction of trials in which the observer reports the signal to be detectable.

This experimental paradigm was adopted in psychophysics at a time when most sensory detection processes were believed to be well-represented by "threshold theory," according to which a stimulus is detected if and only if it exceeds a fixed sensory threshold and false positive reports are ascribed to observer error. Beginning in the early 1950s, threshold theory was challenged and eventually supplanted by statistical decision theory in visual detection tasks (Tanner and Swets, 1954). According to statistical decision theory, visual detection involves a trade-off between the frequencies of true positive and false positive reports, with the balance achieved in an experiment depending upon the particular setting of a critical confidence level or "decision criterion" that the observer chooses to adopt. Thus, the observer can produce virtually any detection rate between zero and 100 percent by setting the decision criterion appropriately. From this perspective, experimental results obtained with the method of constant stimulus are compromised severely by the fact that potential effects of the observer's variable decision criterion are not taken into account; in effect, a potentially important source of variation is not controlled.

An apparent advantage of the method of constant stimulus is that it can be used to determine the dependence of detectability upon any physical parameter of the stimulus (e.g., object or imaging system in image-evaluation studies) in a direct and easily understood way. However, the validity of the method's results depends crucially upon the ability of each observer to hold constant the FPF that would be produced if actually negative trials were presented, and to do so across different imaging conditions — a notoriously difficult task. Clearly, the results depend also upon the observer's ability to resist the temptations of "wishful thinking," in which it is imagined that a virtually invisible stimulus is "seen" because it is known that it is present (Levison and Restle, 1968). In view of these considerations, the method of constant stimulus cannot be recommended generally for the evaluation of image quality.

2.3.3 Diagnostic Accuracy

Many investigators have reported the results of medical tests in terms of the overall percentage of correct diagnoses produced by the test in a mixture of actually positive and actually negative cases. The validity of this index (often called "diagnostic accuracy" in the medical literature) is extremely limited, in part because its numerical value depends strongly on the prevalence of actually positive cases; in part because its value depends upon the observer's setting of his critical confidence level; and in part because it does not reveal the balance of false positive and false negative errors, which can have very different clinical consequences (Metz, 1978).

It should also be noted that some authors, e.g., Swets and Pickett (1982) and Getty et al. (1988), have used the term "diagnostic accuracy" more generally to indicate disease detection performance as measured by ROC analysis and summarized, e.g., by the area under the ROC curve (A_z) index (see Section 4.2.3).

2.3.4 Contrast-Detail Experiments

A "contrast-detail diagram" plots the minimum detectable contrast of an image feature (or signal) as a function of its diameter. Although in principle, different graphs of this kind can be determined with different definitions of "detectability," published contrast-detail diagrams usually have been measured with a "Rose-Burger phantom," in which simple visual signals, such as squares or circles, are present in a single image of a rectangular array such that diameter changes monotonically in each row and contrast changes monotonically in each column (Burger, 1949; 1950; Rose, 1948; 1973), by requiring the observer to state the lowest-contrast signal in each row that is considered detectable.

Although each of the visual stimuli in this kind of experiment is different, the technique suffers from essentially the same limitation as the method of constant stimulus, described previously: its results depend upon the critical confidence level that the observer chooses to adopt, upon the ability to hold a potential — but never measured — FPF constant across stimuli, and upon resistance to "wishful thinking" (Loo et al., 1983). The validity of contrast-detail diagrams measured with a single image of a Rose-Burger phantom is also limited by poor statistical reliability, since each data point is estimated from a single or a few realizations of image noise (Wagner et al., 1985). Therefore, contrast-detail diagrams measured in this way should be used only as a crude exploratory tool in the evaluation of image quality.

2.3.5 Resolution Targets

This is a variant of the contrast-detail experiment. The phantom typically consists of groups of bars, each group with a different spacing and contrast. The observer attempts to determine which groups of bars are resolvable on the image and which are not. The results reflect the resolving capabilities of the imaging system and may be linked to the device resolution as expressed by the LSF and modulation transfer function (see Section 3.2.2). It is important to realize that the summary measure of resolution obtained from bar targets can be a sensitive function of the contrast of the bars when the task is noise limited. The contrast of the bars should, therefore, be specified. The other criticisms of this methodology are the same as those of the contrast-detail approach. The method is, of course, simple and rapid and may thus have a role in day-to-day quality assurance. It is not, however, suitable for fundamental studies of image quality.

2.3.6 Forced Choice Experiments

The problems associated with methods which rely on an absolute internal reference can be overcome by requiring only relative responses from the observer. The simplest form of this type of experiment involves the use of two display areas. At each trial, a known target will be placed in one of the fields and the other will be empty. The observer's task is to identify the field containing the target. This is known as the two-alternative forced choice experiment (Green and Swets, 1966). A multiple-alternative forced-choice experiment involves more display areas, but still only one example of the target (Green and Swets, 1966). The methodology has obvious extensions to discrimination tasks where more than one target type is used. The advantage of the forced-choice paradigm is that experiments are more reproducible and results have an unambiguous interpretation. The method can be criticized as presenting an operating environment which is quite different from clinical practice.

Forced-choice methods have also been used to produce contrast-detail diagrams in which "detectable contrast" is defined rigorously as that contrast (at each signal diameter) which yields a specified percentage of correct responses in an multiple alternative forced-choice experiment. In 18 alternative forced-choice studies reported by Loo et al. (1984), e.g., percentages of correct responses were measured as a function of contrast and the results then interpolated to determine the contrast that would produce 50 percent correct responses.

2.3.7 Graded Response (Receiver Operating Characteristic Curve)

The comments above suggest that there is a need for a test method which deals with the observer's confidence level in a manner which is similar to clinical practice whilst avoiding the problems associated with an internal decision criterion. Graded response experiments fulfill this need. Images are viewed individually and sometimes contain a known target. The observer is asked to grade on a predefined scale his/her degree of certainty that a target is present. The data collected in this way allows an analysis of the trade-off between FPF and TPF yielding the ROC curve, and provides an important insight into clinical cost/benefit. This approach is discussed in detail in Section 4.

2.3.8 Relationship between Graded Response and Method of Constant Stimulus

As shown in Figure 2.1, the relationship between detectability and any imaging parameter can be represented completely by a "three-dimensional" graph in which the axes are true positive response rate, false positive rate and the imaging parameter. A profile through the surface for a constant FPF yields the response curve that would be produced by the method of constant stimulus. Alternatively, a constant value

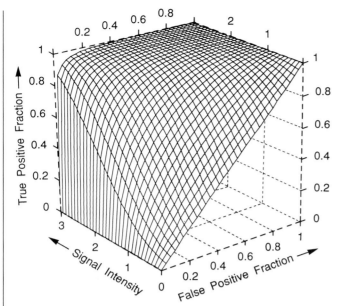

Fig. 2.1. A "three-dimensional" graph in which two-dimensional ROC curves are plotted as a function of signal intensity, thereby generating a surface in three dimensions.

for the imaging parameter produces an ROC curve. Thus, the principal distinctions between these approaches are that the graded response does not readily provide information in terms of the imaging parameter, while the method of constant stimulus takes no cognizance of the changes which can be produced by variations in the decision criteria, *i.e.*, false positive response.

2.4 Summary

As is clear from the above discussion, a variety of approaches exist which are effective in studying specific aspects of imaging system performance. In particular, there is a significant gap between the instrument-based and human-observer based measures of quality, *i.e.*, between the physical and psychophysical. It is the aim of this Report to suggest how image quality can be assessed in such a way that all aspects of the imaging system can be measured in common terms and in a way which is applicable to all types of medical imaging systems.

Of the techniques mentioned above, that of the ideal observer and ROC curve formalisms are the most detailed and exact approaches and will be stressed in this Report. It should, however, be noted that while many of the techniques mentioned above have limitations, they may provide a "rough and ready" technique to identify those aspects of performance which need be studied with greater precision by the proposed approaches.

3. Quality of the Acquired Data

3.1 Introduction

Investigators in the field of signal detection theory have often followed a paradigm, expressed in photographic applications by Shaw and described briefly in Section 1, in which the imaging process is comprised of two stages: detection and display. This was a subtle point in photography, but natural for medical imaging applications, such as CT, where the acquisition of image data is physically, as well as conceptually, a separate step from processing and display of this data (Wagner *et al.*, 1979). The point of view of signal detection theory is that, whereas in the case of display evaluation a detailed understanding of human observers is required, in the case of assessment of the quality of the acquired data, a rigorous ideal observer can be invoked and given a task to perform on the data. The performance of this observer is a unique measure that serves as an upper bound on human or machine observer performance of that task. This performance can be estimated from measurements that are commonly made on imaging systems.

The primary purpose of this Section is to summarize our understanding of ideal-observer performance of imaging tasks. It begins with a review of the analysis of system transfer characteristics and image noise properties upon which much of contemporary image science is based. Next, the fundamentals of signal detection theory are introduced, and the concept of the ideal Bayesian observer is defined. The contribution of the system hardware to the task performance of the Bayesian observer is found to be separable from the specification of the task itself, for some elementary tasks. Finally, several sub-optimal methods of using image data — non-ideal observers — are introduced because they have been found to correlate with human performance for signal detection tasks.

3.2 Physical Performance Measurements

The performance of imaging systems for certain well-specified tasks may be assessed in terms of physical quantities that are typically measured on these systems in the laboratory. The most common of these are the transfer characteristics — the large-area transfer characteristic and the spatial (or detail) transfer characteristic — and the system noise properties. The spatial transfer characteristic typically takes the form of either the PSF or the MTF, and the noise properties are commonly specified by the NPS [also called the Wiener spectrum (W)] or the noise autocovariance function.

The transfer characteristics provide the relationship between objective physical parameters (*e.g.*, x-ray attenuation) and the measured quantities used to generate an image (*e.g.*, optical density or image pixel values). The noise properties measure the corruption of the detected image signal by random fluctuations in the signal and/or the detector. Measurement of these characteristics requires the availability of suitable phantoms and careful attention to their physical composition and its effect on the imaging conditions (*e.g.*, beam hardening in radiography).

The kinds of physical signals generated from objects (phantoms or patients) are treated in Appendix A. Where possible, one defines these signals in such a way that they are intrinsic properties of the object and independent of the imaging conditions. Frequently this can be achieved by working with relative quantities, *e.g.*, the relative activity of neighboring materials or tissues in the radionuclide imaging case. This independence is not always possible, however; in magnetic resonance imaging, the relative signal strengths depend on several time scales characteristic of the imaging technique. In radiography, the signals are dependent on the spectral content of the radiation beam and the energy response of the detector. A calibration technique must be available for controlling such parameters so that the system characterization will be repeatable and readily reproducible in other laboratories.

3.2.1 Large-Area Transfer Characteristics

The simplest large-area transfer characteristic from input to output, *e.g.*, from an input exposure, E, or photon density, Q, to a detector output such as luminance, brightness, or voltage, V, is described by a linear scaling $V = KE$, where K is a constant large-area transfer factor. X-ray image intensifier tubes, gamma cameras and plumbicon camera tubes exhibit such behavior over significant portions of their operating range.

Although this concept may be generalized for non-linear detectors by writing the large-area transfer characteristic as $K(E) = V/E$ at the operating point (E, V) it is then necessary to introduce the incremental-signal transfer factor $\kappa = \Delta V / \Delta E$. In many cases in electronic and photographic imaging, the non-linear dependence can be written locally as a power-law with exponent γ'. Then it is convenient to work in log-log coordinates (Schade, 1951), where γ' becomes the local slope of the linear approximation to the transfer characteristic, *i.e.*,

$$\gamma' = \frac{\Delta(\log V)}{\Delta(\log E)} \qquad (3.1)$$

At the operating point $(\overline{E}, \overline{V})$ at which the slope κ is measured, a simple linear relationship results:

$$\gamma' = \frac{\Delta V/\overline{V}}{\Delta E/\overline{E}} = \frac{\Delta V/\Delta E}{\overline{V}/\overline{E}} = \kappa/\mathrm{K}. \qquad (3.2)$$

Since $\Delta E/\overline{E}$ is the input contrast C_{in} and $\Delta V/\overline{V}$ is the output contrast C_{out}, the quantity $\gamma' = C_{out}/C_{in}$ is simply a contrast gain factor. Therefore, for low-contrast imaging conditions, i.e., small fluctuations about the operating point, a non-linear detection system may be effectively linearized by working on a relative scale, i.e., by using contrast, and using γ' as a contrast transfer or amplification factor.

For photographic and radiographic systems, V refers to film transmission, T. Since density, D, equals the negative logarithm of transmission, one would have

$$\gamma' = \Delta(\log T)/\Delta(\log E) = -\Delta D/\Delta(\log E), \qquad (3.3)$$

which is equal to the conventional radiographic definition of gamma when the negative sign is dropped:

$$\gamma = \Delta D/\Delta(\log E). \qquad (3.4)$$

The minus sign is implicit in the information that a radiograph is a photographic ''negative.''

A set of relationships of great utility in low-contrast analysis of radiographic systems follows from the above definitions:

$$\begin{aligned} \Delta D &= -\Delta(\log T) = -(\log_{10} e)\Delta T/\overline{T} \\ &= \gamma\Delta(\log E) = (\log_{10} e)\gamma \Delta E/\overline{E}. \end{aligned} \qquad (3.5)$$

That is, when one expresses radiographic signals in terms of density differences, ΔD, one is already working on a relative or contrast scale of image brightness (proportional to transmission), and this has a simple relationship to a relative or contrast scale of image exposure. This relative scale will even be found useful for a linear system with gamma of unity. This follows from the fact that by using exposure contrast, i.e., working on a relative exposure scale, physical signals of interest generally become independent of exposure level (e.g., x-ray attenuation, radionuclide uptake). However, it is also common to work with absolute, rather than relative, quantities when a system is linear and the only large-area transfer function that is required is the constant value of K.

Finally, since image luminance and brightness are proportional to film transmission, the definitions of this Section are consistent with the literature of electronic imaging — image tubes, cameras and displays — as well as with the literature of photography and radiography. Note also that the definition of γ (or γ') makes it useful for analyzing a chain of nonlinear components (as in a TV chain): The gamma value of the overall transfer characteristic at a particular operating point is the product of the respective gammas of all component characteristics at that operating point.

3.2.2 Spatial Detail Transfer Characteristics

The discussion above concerned uniform signal changes over a large area. When small areas — or individual detectors — are affected differently by the presence of a structured signal, it is necessary to introduce the detailed system response function, H. This response function describes the way in which the imaging system averages, displaces or blurs input signals, f, before they are detected in the output signal, g. In most general terms, g could be an arbitrary function of f; however, the present treatment is limited to linear (or locally linear) systems, so that the output at some point x_2 in output space is a weighted sum or integral over points x_1 in input space

$$g(x_2) = \int H(x_2, x_1) f(x_1)\, dx_1, \qquad (3.6)$$

or, for the discrete case, in matrix notation (bold lower case for vectors and bold upper case for matrices):

$$\mathbf{g} = \mathbf{Hf}. \qquad (3.7)$$

For simplicity, the inputs and outputs may be considered one dimensional in what follows, with the extension to higher dimensionality being straightforward. Moreover, $\mathbf{g}$ may be thought of as an ''image'' of $\mathbf{f}$, although, in reality, it may be the basic raw data from which an image will be generated, e.g., the projection data from which a CT image could be reconstructed.

The linearity of the system allows for consideration of the image formation process as the ''blurring'' of the input with the system response function, H. For a shift-invariant system, translating the input results simply in a displacement of the output by the same amount (or a simple scaling if magnification is allowed). This implies that H is actually only a function of the difference of coordinates, so that in Equation 3.6, $H(x_1, x_2)$ becomes $H(x_2 - x_1)$, and the equation can then be recognized as the expression used to define a convolution, written in notational shorthand as $g = H * f$. Since, for Fourier transform pairs, a convolution in one domain corresponds to a multiplication in the other, this relationship implies that in the Fourier domain $\tilde{g} = \tilde{H} \cdot \tilde{f}$ ($\tilde{g}$ is the Fourier transform of g, etc.). Reference will be made to linear shift-invariant (LSI) systems in what follows, and it will often be found convenient to work in the Fourier domain for these systems.

A convenient normalization for the system response function H(x) is obtained by requiring its integral over all space to be unity. This means that the total signal intensity, or counts in the case of photon imaging, is preserved under convolution with this function. Under this normalization, the frequency-space representation of the system transfer function in two-dimensional imaging systems is referred to as the optical transfer function (OTF). Quite frequently, its phase is unimportant in elementary signal-detection applications. In that case, the magnitude of the OTF will be used, namely the modulation transfer function (MTF).

In principle, the MTF may be measured in accordance with its definition if one has a set of many sinusoidal test patterns, one for each spatial frequency of interest. One needs to know the modulation or contrast of each test pattern; the pattern is imaged with the modality of interest, and the fraction of modulation or contrast that survives, or is transferred to the image, is recorded. This is the literal implementation of the concept. In most practical cases, the MTF is generated from the image of a line (the LSF) or the image of a point (the PSF) by, respectively, a one-dimensional or a two-dimensional Fourier transformation normalized so that the value of MTF(0) = 1, corresponding to a unit input. The details of implementing this procedure for screen/film systems, together with general mathematical relationships among various techniques independent of modality, are given in ICRU Report 41 (1986). Examples of LSFs and MTFs are given in Figures 3.1 and 3.2.

3.2.3 Elements of System Noise Analysis

In all practical imaging systems, consideration must be given not only to the effect of the transfer characteristics of the imaging system, $\mathbf{g} = \mathbf{Hf}$, but also the corruption of the measurement of $\mathbf{g}$ by the presence of measurement noise. Noise may arise from a number of sources, *e.g.*, photon or thermal fluctuations, and may even be signal dependent. However, for a wide range of practical applications — at least when the signals of interest have low contrast — it is sufficient to consider the measurement noise as additive, that is, signal independent. The imaging equa-

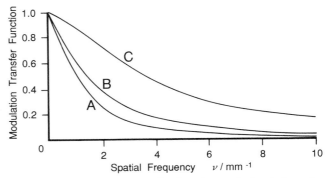

Fig. 3.2. Modulation transfer functions calculated from the measured LSFs of Figure 3.1 (Doi and Rossmann, 1975).

tion is then modified to read

$$\mathbf{g} = \mathbf{Hf} + \mathbf{n} \qquad (3.8)$$

The noise variance is the most common measure of noise. It is inadequate to describe the properties of the noise in the data or image, however, because it does not include the effects of spatial correlation of the noise. For most applications, it is sufficient to consider second-order correlations (ignoring triple correlations among sets of three data points, etc.). Therefore, in what follows, the noise is specified in terms of its mean $\langle n \rangle$ and covariance matrix $\mathbf{C_n}[C_n(i, j) = \langle n(i)n(j) \rangle]$. For additive Gaussian noise, all higher-order statistics are specified for this distribution once the mean and covariance are given (Papoulis, 1965). Usually, one considers zero mean noise. The noise covariance function is said to be stationary when the value of the function depends only on the separation between noise component locations and not on their absolute locations. Hence, only one index is required to describe the noise covariance when stationarity holds.

Usually, the covariance (referred to as the autocovariance in the continuous case) function gives sufficient physical insight into the process responsible for the character of the noise; see, *e.g.*, Figures 3.3 and 3.4. As in the case of transfer function analysis, however, it is frequently easier to work with the frequency-domain content of the noise. One is then interested in characterizing the manner in which the average power of the noise random process is distributed over frequency. When the noise variance is analyzed in terms of its frequency content, one speaks of the noise power spectrum (NPS) or Wiener spectrum, which is written in the continuous case:

$$\mathrm{W_n}(\nu) = \lim_{\mathrm{X} \to \infty} \frac{1}{\mathrm{X}} \left\langle \left| \int_{-\mathrm{X}/2}^{\mathrm{X}/2} \mathrm{dx} \ \mathrm{e}^{-2\pi i \nu x} \mathrm{n(x)} \right|^2 \right\rangle, \qquad (3.9)$$

where the brackets "$\langle \ \rangle$" denote an ensemble average. This conventional definition of the Wiener spectrum refers to a continuous spectral density. It is a function of the continuous spatial frequency variable ν corre-

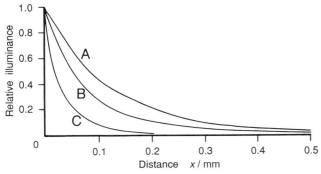

Fig. 3.1. Line spread functions of (A) a fast rare-earth (TRI-MAX), (B) an older calcium tungstate (PAR-RP) and (C) an early mammographic (LO-DOSE) screen-film system (Doi and Rossmann, 1975).

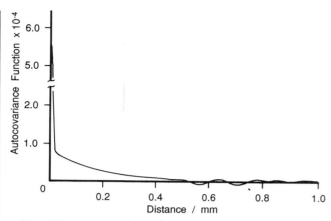

Fig. 3.3. Autocovariance function for a typical screen-film system showing the short-range correlation due to the film grain structure and the long-range correlation due to the scattering of light in the screens (Wagner, 1977a).

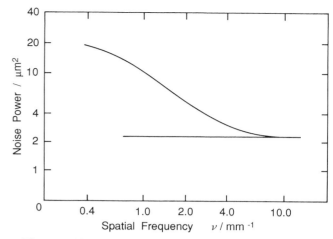

Fig. 3.5. Noise power spectrum for a typical film-screen system exposed to x rays (upper curve) showing quantum mottle and for the film alone exposed to uniform light (lower curve) showing film granularity (corresponding to Figure 3.3).

sponding to the continuous spatial coordinate x. Notational conventions for discrete and continuous representations are given in Appendix C.

It can be shown that for stationary noise, the NPS is the Fourier transform of the autocovariance function (Goodman, 1985). An equivalent statement of this result is that the noise covariance matrix is diagonalized by a Fourier transformation when the noise is stationary (Andrews and Hunt, 1977). Examples of noise power spectra corresponding to the autocovariance functions of Figures 3.3 and 3.4 are given in Figures 3.5 and 3.6.

Image artifacts are another source of system performance degradation; they are not considered here, but are discussed further in Section 5.

3.2.3.1 Pre- and Post-Noise Insertion Processes. A transfer function $\mathbf{H}'$ may act on noise as well as on the input signal, giving $\mathbf{n}' = \mathbf{H}'\mathbf{n}$. For the case of a noise process that is filtered or "colored" with a transfer function $\tilde{H}'(\nu)$ to produce a new noise

process, the new NPS, $W'(\nu)$ becomes

$$W'(\nu) = W(\nu)|\tilde{H}'(\nu)|^2.$$

The transfer function is referred to as a post-noise-insertion transfer. That is, the new noise process is derived from linear combinations of the original process. This happens, for example, when a noise process is acted upon by an image processing algorithm or the ideal-observer discrimination algorithms described below.

On the other hand, when a system component has a transfer function that filters the mean signal without coloring the noise, the transfer function is referred to as "pre-noise-insertion." This means that the transfer function that governs the mean image has no effect on the final noise correlations. There are many common realizations of this phenomenon; *e.g.*, a

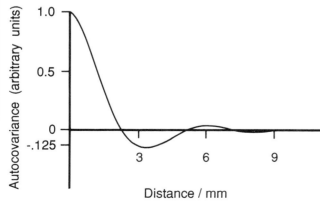

Fig. 3.4. Normalized autocovariance function for the first generation CT system showing the negative correlation (near 3 mm) induced by the subtractions inherent to CT algorithms (Wagner and Sandrick, 1979).

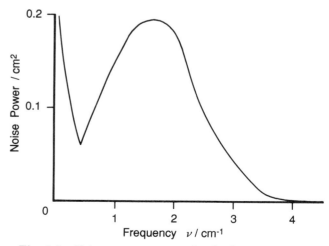

Fig. 3.6. Noise power spectrum for the first generation CT (corresponding to Figure 3.4). The low-frequency artifact has not yet been removed from this result (see Section 5.3.3.1) (Wagner *et al.*, 1979).

gamma-camera collimator blurs the mean radionuclide image without altering the Poisson (uncorrelated) nature of the detection process.

3.3 Bayesian Signal Detection Theory and the Ideal Observer

If one has the measurements of the large area (or macroscopic) transfer characteristic, the spatial detail transfer function, or MTF, and the NPS at the operating point of interest for an imaging system under study, the performance of the imaging system can be predicted for a special observer, the ideal observer of Bayesian signal detection theory. The ideal observer is the Bayesian decision maker who minimizes the "cost" or "risk" when determining a decision strategy for a given task. This observer calculates a ratio of likelihoods or probabilities for two competing hypotheses and decides in favor of the most probable hypothesis as weighted by the cost and prevalence ratios. This is called a likelihood-ratio decision strategy (see Appendix C).

The ideal-observer formalism is applicable to many imaging tasks; however, it is most easily applied to a special category of tasks referred to as the signal-known-exactly/background-known-exactly (SKE/BKE) case. The SKE/BKE task is one in which a completely specified signal is to be detected against a completely specified background, or two such signals on the same known background are to be discriminated. In clinical terms, this refers to images in which all the details about the lesion, its location, size, shape, etc., as well as all the features of the anatomical background, are known by the clinician. The hypotheses then refer only to whether the image includes the lesion or not.

Appendix C describes in detail the strategy used by the ideal observer to minimize the probability of making an incorrect decision when classifying a given data vector. For an SKE/BKE task, it is shown that the ideal observer's strategy is simply to undo any correlations in the image noise by "whitening" its spectrum, and then apply a filter matched to the expected difference signal. This observer is therefore called the prewhitening matched filter (PWMF). The output of the ideal observer's filtering of the data is a decision variable (see Figure 1.2). The classification of a particular data vector is determined by whether the decision variable falls above or below the observer's criterion for separating the classes. The ideal-observer SNR, or SNR_I, is a measure of the overlap of the decision variable outcomes that would be obtained for the ensemble of data vectors in the two classes.

For the SKE/BKE case, the decision maker is given the image data set g, and must decide which of two objects, f_1 or f_2, is most compatible with this data set. The objects are known and non-random, so the only fluctuations in the data are due to noise. If the noise is also assumed to be stationary, then it is usually more convenient to work in the spatial-frequency domain with the (inherently diagonal) NPS rather than in the spatial domain with the autocovariance function. Therefore, the equations which are presented in this Section will be in the spatial-frequency domain, where $\tilde{f}_i$ is the Fourier transform of the object present under hypothesis i, $\Delta\tilde{f}$ is the Fourier-domain difference object ($\Delta\tilde{f} = \tilde{f}_2 - \tilde{f}_1$), and $\tilde{H} = K\,OTF$, where OTF is the optical transfer function, whose magnitude is the modulation transfer function (MTF).

It is shown in Appendix C that the figure of merit for the ideal decision maker for a simple hypothesis-testing task is:

$$SNR_I^2 = K^2 \int \frac{|\tilde{f}(\nu)|^2\, MTF^2(\nu)}{W_n(\nu)}\, d\nu = d'^2_{SKE}, \quad (3.10)$$

where W_n is the noise power spectrum. d'_{SKE} is the detectability index for the SKE/BKE situation. Other subscripts and superscripts are used with the symbol d depending upon the type of observer and method of obtaining the index, as explained in Section 4.2.3. For situations where it is not appropriate to work in the spatial-frequency domain, the SNR can be calculated in the spatial domain (see Appendix C).

A number of examples demonstrating the application of the ideal observer to medical imaging are given in Appendix D.

3.4 Spatial-Frequency Dependence of Ideal Observer SNR

The practical importance and general utility of the concept embodied in Equation 3.10 will be explained here using straightforward manipulations of that expression. This will provide the motivation and facilitate the understanding of its applicability to design, evaluation and optimization of imaging systems.

The notation in this Report generally follows the common convention of the imaging equation, Equation 3.8, $g = Hf + n$, where f is the input and the detected data is g. For the present Section, however, a notation that is symmetric between input and output will be adopted. Quantities referred to the input will here be distinguished from those referred to the output by subscripts "in" or "out." For example, the parameter $\Delta\tilde{f}$ elsewhere in the Report implicitly carries the subscript "in." Here that quantity will be labelled $\Delta\tilde{f}_{in}$ to distinguish it from the same quantity referred to the output, namely $\Delta\tilde{f}_{out}$. The latter would be noted $\Delta\tilde{g}$ in the convention of the imaging equation; a symmetric notation is adopted and expanded upon here. The purpose of the more elaborate notation is to motivate and simplify the introduction of the equations commonly encountered in Ideal Observer analysis of imaging systems.

3.4.1 Task Factor and Physical Measurements Factor

First, notice that the factors in the numerator of Equation 3.10 could be combined to define an effective output signal "power":

$$|\Delta \tilde{f}_{out}(\nu)|^2 \equiv K^2 |\Delta \tilde{f}_{in}(\nu)|^2 MTF^2(\nu) \qquad (3.11)$$

The quantity $\Delta \tilde{f}(\nu)$ of Equation 3.10 is written here as $\Delta \tilde{f}_{in}(\nu)$. The quantity $W_n(\nu)$ of Equation 3.9, which bears the subscript n because it is the spectrum of the noise n, is referred to here as $W_{out}(\nu)$ since it is measured at the output. The expanded notation allows the SNR^2_I of Equation 3.10 to be written

$$SNR^2_I = \int \frac{|\Delta \tilde{f}_{out}(\nu)|^2}{W_{out}(\nu)} d\nu \qquad (3.12)$$

where the numerator and denominator are both in terms of output quantities. Alternatively, one could write

$$SNR^2_I = \int \frac{|\Delta \tilde{f}_{in}(\nu)|^2}{W_{in}(\nu)} d\nu \qquad (3.13)$$

where the system measurements K, $MTF(\nu)$ and $W_{out}(\nu)$ have been combined into the quantity $W_{in}(\nu)$:

$$\frac{1}{W_{in}(\nu)} = \frac{K^2 MTF^2(\nu)}{W_{out}(\nu)} \qquad (3.14)$$

and the numerator and denominator of the SNR expression are both effectively in terms of input quantities. $W_{in}(\nu)$ is seen to be the output noise power, $W_{out}(\nu)$, referred—through the system transfer characteristics—to the input. It is defined in terms of its inverse, rather than directly, because it is generally encountered in this form, and is well-behaved: it may have zeros, but it will not have singularities. Equation 3.13 has the advantage that the task—as described by $|\Delta \tilde{f}_{in}(\nu)|^2$—may be separated from the performance of the system hardware—as described by $1/W_{in}(\nu)$. The latter factor is independent of the task. This separation is not possible with Equation 3.12.

The quantities that make up the numerator and denominator of the factor K, respectively the output variable and input variable at the operating point of interest, can be used to normalize the other factors in Equation 3.10, allowing relative quantities, or contrasts, to be used instead of absolute quantities. Thus one may write

$$SNR^2_I = \int \frac{|(\Delta \tilde{f}_{in}(\nu))_{rel}|^2 MTF^2(\nu)}{(W_{out}(\nu))_{rel}} d\nu \qquad (3.15)$$

where the subscript "rel" means normalized by its mean value: Δf is normalized by the mean input quantity, and the output variable in W_{out} is normalized by the mean output value.

All of this is strictly rigorous for a linear detection system. Now, suppose that the detection system is nonlinear. Then a small-signal approximation may be made with κ replacing K. Since $\kappa = \gamma' K = -\gamma K$, one arrives once more at Equation 3.15, but with an additional factor γ^2 in the numerator. That is,

$$SNR^2_I = \int \frac{|(\Delta \tilde{f}_{in}(\nu))_{rel}|^2 \gamma^2 MTF^2(\nu)}{(W_{out}(\nu))_{rel}} d\nu \qquad (3.16)$$

In the language of Section 3.2.1, a non-linear detection system has been effectively linearized by working on a relative scale, i.e., by working in terms of contrast, and using γ or (γ') as a contrast amplification factor.

3.4.2 Definitions of NEQ and DQE

Consider, for example, the case of radiographic screen-film imaging where the output NPS is specified in terms of fluctuations of relative transmission, $\Delta T/T$. Then we may write for the inverse of $(W_{in})_{rel}$:

$$\begin{aligned} \frac{1}{(W_{in})_{rel}} &= \frac{\gamma^2 MTF^2(\nu)}{W_{\Delta T/T}(\nu)} \\ &= \frac{(\log_{10} e)^2 \gamma^2 MTF^2(\nu)}{W_{\Delta D}(\nu)} \equiv NEQ(\nu) \end{aligned} \qquad (3.17)$$

This expression defines the spectrum of noise equivalent quanta, $NEQ(\nu)$, and allows one to write

$$SNR^2_I = \int |(\Delta \tilde{f}_{in}(\nu))_{rel}|^2 NEQ(\nu) d\nu \qquad (3.18)$$

The quantity $NEQ(\nu)$ can be interpreted as the number of quanta at the input of a perfect detector that would yield the same output noise, as a function of spatial frequency, as the real detection system under consideration. The quantity γ appearing in this expression must have the same output units as those used in the measurement of $W_{\Delta T/T}$ or $W_{\Delta D}$. That is, if the NPS is measured in terms of diffuse (or specular) transmission or density, then γ must be measured in terms of diffuse (or specular) transmission or density. As noted above, the analysis presented here treats all inputs and outputs as one-dimensional. Details of the extension of such frequency domain analysis to two or more dimensions are treated by Dainty and Shaw (1974) and Metz and Doi (1979).

The concept of $NEQ(\nu)$ serves several purposes. It represents a unique quotient of system measurements that enter into the calculation of the performance of the ideal observer. It also serves the practical purpose of transforming noise power measurements made in terms of output quantities that may be arbitrary or peculiar to a particular measurement system, e.g., specular density, digital pixel intensity numbers, etc., to an input quantity that has universal and therefore portable interpretation, *e.g.*, photon density (or its inverse, as in the application to image intensifier tubes or gamma cameras given in Appendix D).

The frequency dependence given by W_{in} or NEQ summarizes the contribution of the imaging system hardware working at a particular operating point (exposure, density, time, etc.) to the performance of the task by the ideal observer. The frequency dependence of the task determines the relative importance of regions in frequency space for the task performance, and provides the weighting of the imaging system response in the overall measure of the ideal-observer performance given by Equation 3.13 or Equation 3.18.

Although first defined for photographic imaging (Shaw, 1963), NEQ is in fact a particular case of a more general form encountered frequently in information theory (Shaw, 1963; Dainty and Shaw, 1974; Shaw, 1978), signal detection theory (Whalen, 1971; Wagner and Brown, 1985) and elsewhere throughout applications in communications engineering. Because of the existing terminology, later authors often refer to a quotient of the form W_{in}^{-1} ($\mathbf{H^t C_n^{-1} H}$ of the Appendices) as the NEQ factor even when the input units are different from those of the conventional NEQ (counts per unit area) (see, *e.g.*, Myers *et al.*, 1990; Barrett *et al.*, 1994). It is the structure, not necessarily the units, that is being identified as a general concept broadly applicable to linear, or linearizable, imaging systems. When the concept and units are used literally, it means that the system has been linearized for relative signals or contrast and photon-limited images. Then the factor representing the task, $\Delta\tilde{f}(\nu)$, must also be measured or specified in terms of relative signals or contrast. Otherwise, an absolute scale is required. In either case it is essential that the transfer characteristics and the noise measurements correspond to the same beam quality, pulse sequence and/or other physical parameters that determine the signal strength.

Measurements and analysis of image data in terms of the NEQ(ν) spectrum have been carried out for a wide range of applications: photography, electronic imaging and unconventional imaging systems (Shaw, 1963; 1978); CT (Wagner *et al.*, 1979; Hanson, 1979a; 1979b; Borasi *et al.*, 1984); radiography (Fisher, 1982); magnification radiography (Sandrick and Wagner, 1982); gamma camera imaging (Grossman *et al.*, 1984; 1986); and mammography (Wagner and Muntz, 1979; Nishiyama and Yaffe, 1985; Bunch *et al.*, 1987; Bunch, 1989). An example from CT is given in Figure 3.7. In this case the density of counts is per unit length along the circumference of the slice; the slice thickness has been integrated out (see Appendix D). Once the NEQ spectrum is measured, it may be compared with the actual level of exposure quanta required to make the image. This comparison leads to

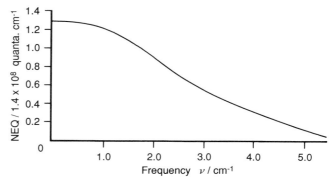

Fig. 3.7. Noise equivalent quanta for a second generation CT scanner.

the concept of detective quantum efficiency (DQE) and this is discussed, together with examples, in Appendix D. The dependence of NEQ and DQE on exposure level (or analogous parameters that define an operating point in other modalities) allows for a quantitative determination of the dynamic range, and this is also exemplified in Appendix D. If the image detail of interest modifies the shape of the energy spectrum, as in the imaging of bone or iodine, a more general approach may be required (Tapiovaara and Wagner, 1985).

3.4.3 Elementary Detection and Discrimination Tasks

To illustrate how the task factor f and the hardware response NEQ combine to determine detectability, two examples of elementary tasks are considered, as shown in Figures 3.8 and 3.9. Task 1 is illustrated in Figure 3.8, where the two-dimensional intensity distribution of a Gaussian-shaped lesion on a flat background is shown. This is f_2. The flat (signal absent) background is f_1. The template is then the difference between these two and corresponds to the distribution of intensity in the figure.

Task 2 is a more complicated "resolution" task. It is illustrated in Figure 3.9, where the two-dimen-

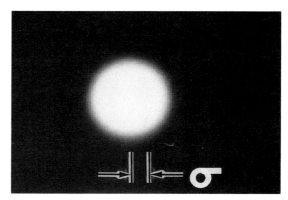

Fig. 3.8. The single lesion, low-frequency task: The detection of a Gaussian lesion against a uniform background.

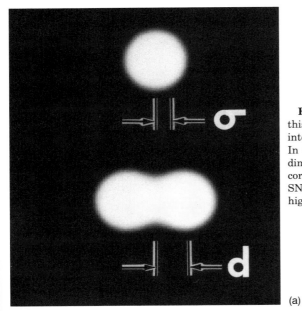

(a)

Fig. 3.9. Mid- to high-frequency task: as shown in (a) the two hypotheses for this task are that the image is of a single lesion, or of two lesions each of half the intensity of the single one, separated by some finite distance (Wagner *et al.*, 1985). In (b) the solid and dashed lines show the two alternative hypotheses, in one dimension, and the dotted line the difference between these curves. In (c) the corresponding power spectra, which determine the relative contributions to the $SNR_I{}^2$, are plotted. This demonstrates the increased significance of the mid- to high-frequency components in the signals for this task (Hanson, 1983).

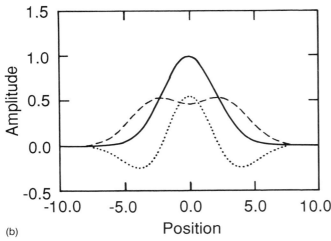

(b)

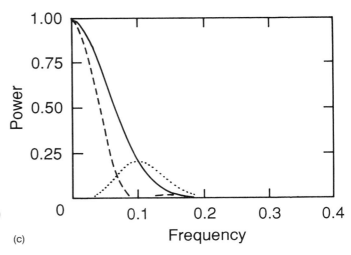

(c)

sional intensity distribution of two lesions separated by some finite distance is shown. One hypothesis, H_2, is that two lesions are present; the other, H_1, is that only a single lesion of double intensity is present. Then Δf is the difference between the double-lesion and the single-lesion intensity distributions, and the profile of this difference along the direction of separation is shown in Figure 3.9b. It is instructive to consider these tasks in the spatial-frequency domain. The difference signal of Task 1 is represented by the Gaussian frequency spectrum shown in Figure 3.9c (solid line). The spectrum of Task 2 is also shown in Figure 3.9c (dotted line). Task 1 is referred to as a low-frequency task and Task 2 as a band-pass task. Tasks of Type 1 will tend to place greater weight on the zero- and low-frequency portion of the $NEQ(\nu)$ response. However, there are many tasks where the expected background level is not known or must be estimated — more typical of clinical situations. These tasks are akin to Task 2 and will tend to place greater

weight on the mid- and higher-frequency portions of the $NEQ(\nu)$ spectrum.

If measurements of all of the quantities that enter into Equations 3.13 and 3.18 are obtained at the same system operating point and imaging conditions, they may be combined to yield an estimate of the SNR_I, the upper bound on the performance of the specified task by any observer. Some alternative observers are introduced below. These are model observers that have been used either to approximate the ideal observer or to approximate the human observer for certain classes of tasks. Estimates of the performance of these observers may frequently be obtained by implementing them using machine (computer) algorithms.

3.5 Non-Ideal Observers

Besides the ideal observer, there are other model observers that are of interest in imaging system performance evaluation. This is particularly the case when task complexity precludes straightforward calculation of the ideal-observer performance and/or when an observer more closely aligned with human performance is desired. Two such observers are the Hotelling and non-prewhitening matched filter observers.

3.5.1 The Hotelling Observer

When the signal or background are only known statistically, the SNR_I may not be calculable or may require lengthy numerical calculations using Monte Carlo simulations (Brown and Insana, 1988). Moreover, the strategy employed by the ideal observer in such cases is generally non-linear (Wagner *et al.*, 1989), and it is unclear whether human observers can perform non-linear operations on the data. So for medical imaging systems that will have human observers as the end-users, it may be desirable to use model observers that are more tractable and that more faithfully reflect the capabilities of the human observer, specifically the class of linear observers.

The Hotelling observer (Hotelling, 1931) demonstrates maximum discrimination ability among all observers that are limited to performing only linear operations on the data. In spite of the linear limitation, this approach provides a formalism for determining separability between data from two hypothesized states when the objects to be detected or discriminated have variability. The Hotelling approach has been previously described for the specific problem of image assessment in medical imaging by Barrett (Barrett *et al.*, 1985; Barrett, 1990).

In Appendix E, it is shown that in the spatial-frequency domain the SNR for the Hotelling observer is given by:

$$SNR_{Hot}^2 = \int \frac{|\Delta \bar{\tilde{f}}(\nu)|^2 |\tilde{H}(\nu)|^2}{W_g(\nu)} \, d\nu \qquad (3.19)$$

The difference object spectrum, $\Delta \bar{\tilde{f}}(\nu)$, in this expression is the difference between the spectra of the average objects under each of the hypotheses. $W_g(\nu)$ is the Fourier transform of the average overall covariance of the data. It contains a term corresponding to object variability as well as the term corresponding to the usual measurement noise. The Fourier representation is only valid when the overall covariance function is stationary and the imaging system is linear and shift invariant. Otherwise, the Hotelling figure of merit must be evaluated in the space domain (see Appendix E).

3.5.2 The Non-Prewhitening Matched Filter (NPWMF)

The NPWMF is a sub-optimal observer in that, while it uses all known information regarding the signal parameters perfectly, unlike the ideal observer of Section 3.3 it is unable to undo any correlations in the data, or weight in favor of less noisy dimensions. Thus, it has a lower discrimination ability than that of the ideal observer in situations where the noise is colored, *i.e.*, where the Wiener spectrum is frequency dependent. Interest in this sub-optimal observer stems from several studies of human discrimination performance that suggest that the NPWMF is a better predictor of human performance than the ideal observer for SKE/BKE tasks in which the noise is correlated (Burgess *et al.*, 1981; Myers *et al.*, 1985). In addition, for more complicated tasks, where either the signal or the background has some variability (specified in a statistical manner), it is often easier to calculate the NPWMF figure of merit than that of the ideal observer (Myers *et al.*, 1990).

Just as for the ideal and Hotelling SNRs, the Fourier representation of the SNR for the NPWMF observer, SNR_{npw}, can be written in terms of the NPS and the MTF of the system, provided that the noise is stationary and the imaging system is linear and shift invariant. When the object has some variability, the object autocovariance must also be stationary for the Fourier domain expression to be meaningful. As shown in Appendix F:

$$SNR_{npw}^2 = \frac{[\int |\Delta \bar{\tilde{f}}(\nu)|^2 |\tilde{H}(\nu)|^2 \, d\nu]^2}{\int |\Delta \bar{\tilde{f}}(\nu)|^2 |\tilde{H}(\nu)|^2 \, W_g(\nu) \, d\nu} , \qquad (3.20)$$

where $W_g(\nu)$ is the total effective noise power in the data. This Fourier representation is valid only when stationary statistics apply, which generally requires the signal to be of low contrast. For Poisson noise at high contrasts, the denominator must be computed in the space domain (see Appendix F).

A practical modification of the NPWMF has been suggested by Tapiovaara and Wagner (1993). This modified NPWMF, referred to as the DC-suppressing observer, has a strategy identical to the NPWMF, except for the fact that it doesn't consider mean image brightness. It thereby ignores both the signal and the noise in the zero-frequency channel. This modification is motivated by the fact that the human visual response is known to be low at very low frequencies (Van Nes and Bouman, 1967), by the evidence that humans cannot use absolute image brightness as a useful image feature for detection (Ratliff, 1965; Rolland *et al.*, 1991), and by the observation that the variation in DC level of electronic imaging systems would significantly degrade the performance of the NPWMF (Tapiovaara, 1993), yet would be almost unnoticed by the human observer. The performance of this observer should, therefore, more closely approximate the human observer than does the non-prewhitening matched filter.

3.5.3 Experimental Implementation of Model Observers

If there is sufficient time, and it is otherwise practical to obtain a large number of phantom images, it is possible to implement non-ideal observers in practice and measure the SNRs directly (Tapiovaara and Wagner, 1993). One requires a phantom appropriate to each of the two hypotheses to be discriminated. A large number of images for each hypothesis are collected and averaged to render the noise negligible; the difference template corresponding to the observer's decision strategy can then be constructed and stored; and finally this template is applied to a large number of images for both hypothesis states. The means and variances of the decision function output can then be measured and the appropriate SNR calculated by the simple expression of Equation C.5, which finds the squared difference of the means in units of the average variance. This approach may require a check that the noise is additive and Gaussian, but requires no other model of the imaging system or its performance characteristics. For widespread utility, it requires only consensus on the composition of the test patterns for various practical hypotheses.

3.6 Relationship between Signal-to-Noise Ratio and Performance of Ideal and Quasi-Ideal Observers

The SNR figures of merit are directly related to the ROC curve discussed in detail in Section 4. Signal-to-noise ratio is abbreviated as d' to simplify writing the error integrals below and to conform to traditional usage. The probability distributions for the decision function under the two hypotheses are shown in Figure 3.10. Note that in units of the standard deviation, the difference in the means is just the "distance," SNR = d'.

One can now calculate the probabilities of a true-positive decision and a false-positive decision when the decision function is distributed as shown in Figure 3.10. One can deduce from that figure the

result for the true positive rate, p(TP),

$$p(TP) = (2\pi)^{-1/2} \int_{C-(d'/2)}^{\infty} dx \; e^{-x^2/2}, \quad (3.21)$$

where C is the decision or threshold criterion. Similarly the false positive rate p(FP) is given by:

$$p(FP) = (2\pi)^{-1/2} \int_{C+(d'/2)}^{\infty} dx \; e^{-x^2/2}. \quad (3.22)$$

When the decision criterion is varied, the resulting p(TP) and p(FP) levels trace out the ROC curve.

For the ideal observer, the quantity d' is referred to as the detectability index, d'_{SKE}. It is the SNR for the ideal (Bayesian) observer for performing the task of differentiating between two hypotheses when the signals and backgrounds are known exactly (SKE/BKE). Other subscripts and superscripts are used with the symbol d' depending on the type of observer and the method of obtaining the index. For example, when the index is derived *a posteriori* from the area under the ROC curve (see Section 4.2.3), the index d_a is used, and is not limited to the equal variance case being treated here (*e.g.*, it could be the Hotelling SNR). In the context of signal detection in additive Gaussian noise, the SNR is now seen to serve as a limit on the error integrals that determine performance.

3.7 Comparing the Ideal and the Human Observer

A study of the correlation between human visual performance and the predictions of model observer SNRs has been carried out by Loo *et al.* (1984) for the task of detecting low-contrast beads. It was found that SNRs based on the NPWMF observer gave an excellent correlation with human visual performance if a human visual transfer function was introduced into both numerator and denominator (the PWMF and NPWMF also gave excellent agreement with the human). In addition, Ishida *et al.* (1984) and Giger and Doi (1985; 1987) have shown that detection tasks using simple square objects and human observers can be predicted if a term representing the internal visual noise is incorporated into this model. Related investigations and results have been reported by deBelder *et al.* (1971) and Wolf (1980). Giger and Doi (1984; 1985; 1987) and Giger *et al.* (1984) showed how the effects of sampling and aliasing in digital systems could be successfully incorporated into such model observers. A "channelized" ideal observer — lacking the infinitely fine frequency resolution of the PWMF — was found to correlate highly with human observer performance while remaining indistinguishable from the NPWMF in performance (Myers and Barrett, 1987). More recently, the Hotelling observer modified to operate through spatial-frequency-selective channels was found to predict human perfor-

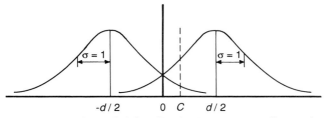

Fig. 3.10. The probability distributions corresponding to the two hypotheses. They have a standard deviation equal to unity and are separated by a distance of d' standard deviations. C is the decision criterion being used.

mance for tasks with both human variability and anti-correlated noise (Barrett *et al.*, 1993). For a more detailed summary of human observer studies in the context of signal detection theory, see the major review by Chesters (1992), and further discussion in Appendix G.

3.7.1 Statistical Efficiency

Tanner and Birdsall (1958) suggested that human sensory performance be assessed by comparing human results to those of an ideal observer performing the same task, and that this comparison be described by the term "statistical efficiency." [Compare the general concept of statistical efficiency (Whalen, 1971).] Two definitions of statistical efficiency have been used, one based on detectability indices and the other based on SNRs of the stimuli on which the detection process is based. Respectively, these definitions are:

$$\text{F}_1 = \left\{\frac{d'_{\text{H}}}{d'_{\text{I}}}\right\}^2 , \quad \text{F}_2 = \left\{\frac{\text{SNR}_{\text{I}}}{\text{SNR}_{\text{R}}}\right\}^2 , \qquad (3.23)$$

where d'_{H} and d'_{I} are the values of the detectability index d' achieved by the human observer and ideal observer in performing the same specified task, and SNR_{R} and SNR_{I} are the physical SNRs of the stimulus that are required by the real and ideal observers to perform the task at the same level. The two definitions are equivalent if d' is linearly proportional to the physical SNR of the stimulus. There are some situations where this proportionality does not hold for human observers. Although Tanner and Birdsall defined the efficiency F_1 in terms of the detectability index d', this only applies to normally distributed decision functions. This efficiency can be defined more generally in terms of d_{a} (see Section 4.3.2).

Barlow (1978; 1980) measured efficiency for the detection of random dot patterns and obtained results in the vicinity of 50 percent. Burgess *et al.* (1981) extended this to amplitude discrimination of simple test patterns in gray-scale images and found efficiencies above 50 percent. Similar results have been reported by Watson *et al.* (1984) for noiseless sine waves and by Kersten and Barlow (1984). Burgess and Ghandeharian (1984a) also found efficiencies of 50 percent for a more complicated task involving signal location uncertainty. Markedly lower efficiencies have been reported for detection tasks on anticorrelated noise backgrounds (Myers *et al.*, 1985) and for texture discrimination tasks (Wagner *et al.*, 1990a).

3.7.2 Sources of Human Inefficiency

It is likely that there are a number of sources of human inefficiency (Wilcox, 1968; Pelli, 1985). Humans may not use exactly the correct expected signal function for the correlation process (*i.e.*, the correct "matching filter") or they might not be able to use the location information precisely. The observer may have some "internal noise" due to variability in the conversion from a physical correlation scale to a sensory visibility scale; this is usually ascribed to neural noise (Barlow, 1957), but can be caused also by decision-variable fluctuations (Wickelgreen, 1968; Burgess and Colborne, 1988). There may also be incomplete collection and weighting of image data. Finally, the human may not be able to set a completely stable decision criterion. A fuller discussion of the efficiency of the human observer is given in Appendix G.

3.8 Estimation

The generalization of the signal detection or classification paradigm from the task of choosing the most likely of two signals to that of selecting the most likely of the universe of signals is called estimation and plays a critical role in contemporary quantitative image analysis. When the entire universe of signals serve as candidates for the estimation process, we speak of estimation with no *a priori* knowledge of parameters of the candidate signals. In this case, the most commonly used estimation scheme is referred to as maximum likelihood estimation, which — when the noise is additive and Gaussian — reduces to simple inverse filtering of the image data (if the inverse, H^{-1} of the system matrix exists). The technique is discussed in many texts (*e.g.*, Whalen, 1971) and the resulting estimates have statistical properties similar to those found for likelihood functions.

The next level of estimation involves having a model or probability distribution of the class of objects expected in the image. A common technique for this is maximum *a posteriori* (MAP) estimation; one maximizes the *a posteriori* probability of a given object using a prior model of the objects to be expected, together with the conditional probability for the actual data given a particular object. Several authors (Hanson, 1987; Barrett, 1986; Andrews and Hunt, 1977) have pointed out that many commonly used estimation techniques can be understood in terms of MAP estimation.

Barrett has recently given an elaborate development of the relationship between figures of merit for detection or classification and figures of merit for estimation (Barrett, 1990) for the case of linear classifiers and estimators. It is clear from that work that unambiguous objective quantitative assessment of imaging system performance can be carried out once the task is clearly specified, at least for linear procedures. Müller *et al.* (1990), Hanson (1990), and Myers and Hanson (1990; 1991) have given numerical procedures based on task performance for nonlinear procedures. Rigorous formulations of the problem of image assessment for image reconstruction and restoration algorithms are in progress. It is clear that they will depend on the task that the imaging system faces and that they will involve rigorous statistical assessment of the algorithm under independent repeated trials.

A more detailed discussion of estimation and the errors associated with estimation tasks is given in Appendix H.

3.9 Summary

Some fundamentals of contemporary image science have been presented in this Section. The analysis began with the basic physical descriptors of imaging system performance: the large-area transfer characteristic, the detail transfer function, and several measures of system noise properties. The noise covariance matrix and its continuous counterpart, the noise autocovariance function, were studied since these completely characterize the zero-mean Gaussian noise that reasonably approximates the fluctuations in image data of many common physical imaging processes.

The Bayesian ideal observer strategy was described here and is given in detail in Appendix C. The performance of this observer on the SKE/BKE task of detection of completely specified signals against completely specified background (or the discrimination between two such signals) may be rigorously quantified. The ideal observer uses prior knowledge of the kinds of signals to be detected or discriminated and the detected image data to calculate the betting odds for or against the presence of the signal (or between the signals to be discriminated). This observer performs an operation on the detected data that is equivalent to decorrelating the noise in the data — known as prewhitening — and then matched filters to the expected difference signal between the alternatives. The observer is therefore called the matched filter or the prewhitening matched filter. The output of the filter is used as a decision variable which is then compared to a threshold to yield the decision for or against the signal (or between the alternatives). The performance of the Bayesian observer is straightforward to calculate since it is a special linear filter. The SNR achieved by this filter completely determines the performance of the ideal observer for such tasks. In fact, the ROC curve is readily generated from an elementary error function whose argument includes the SNR and the decision threshold.

This Bayesian SNR_I includes two fundamental factors. The first is a combination of the fundamental imaging measurements on the imaging system hardware, namely the transfer characteristics and the NPS at the operating point of interest. This combination was shown to be equivalent to a reflection or scaling of the measurement noise back to the domain of the object or incoming radiation. For applications where relative signals, *e.g.*, contrast, are measured, the combination is interpreted as the number of quanta, or NEQ, the image is worth at that operating point. The second factor is independent of the imaging system and characterizes the task required of the observer. In the frequency domain, the SNR is simply a task-weighted combination of the SNRs available from the hardware at each spatial frequency.

For more complicated tasks, *e.g.*, when signal variability is allowed, the Bayesian observer does not generally take a simple linear form. There are, however, two sub-optimal observers that have been found to correlate with human observers for such tasks. The first is the Hotelling or best linear observer, a generalization of the matched filter that uses the complete class variability to generate a template that matches to the average difference between the classes to be discriminated, and against the total noise. The second is the NPWMF, an observer that is unable to prewhiten the noise, but otherwise forms the appropriate template before decision making.

In this Section and the related appendices, problems of image estimation and reconstruction have been cast in Bayesian terms using the likelihood function and estimates of prior and posterior probability distributions. Figures of merit for estimation problems can, as noted in Appendix H, be derived from the Fisher Information Matrix, which, in the case of additive Gaussian noise, takes a form that includes the system measurement matrix, a generalization of the NEQ concept. Ambiguity exists concerning figures of merit for image estimation problems when the task that the image is to serve is not specified; however, it is clear that the system measurement matrix plays a fundamental role in Bayesian image performance assessment.

Great progress has been made in the quantitative evaluation of imaging systems through the use of concepts from Fourier optics and statistical decision theory. However, the required physical performance measurements may require a substantial effort, as will the determination of their uncertainties. Further work is continuing to extend these ideas to areas such as more complicated and realistic imaging tasks and to problems such as those presented by image artifacts.

4. Quality of the Observed Image

4.1 The Need for an Empirical Approach to Image Quality

At present, and in the foreseeable future, diagnostic images must be interpreted by human observers. Therefore, image quality in medicine must be judged in terms of the extent to which a class of images allows real observers, such as radiologists, to correctly determine each patient's state of health or disease. Although image quality in this practical sense may be inferred, in some cases, from the calculated performance of an ideal observer (see Section 3), final judgements concerning image quality must, at least for the present, be made empirically, by measuring human observer performance directly.

4.2 Receiver Operating Characteristic (ROC) Analysis

For simplicity, the evaluation of observer performance is usually restricted to situations in which possible truth concerning the object can be divided into two states (e.g., "abnormal" vs. "normal," "malignancy present" vs. "malignancy absent," etc.) and in which two corresponding decisions can be made. The adequacy and limitations of this restriction are discussed elsewhere (Metz, 1986a; 1988). Often, the two states are indicated by the abstract terms "positive" and "negative" to denote a defined (possibly composite) truth state and its complement. In studies that seek to measure medical image quality, the two states of truth can be chosen by the designer of the experiment to represent alternative diagnoses, the presence and absence of some diagnostically relevant image feature, or the presence and absence of an idealized geometric object. Images obtained from actual clinical cases, phantoms or computer simulation can be used in the experiment, depending on the compromise between realism and convenience that is considered appropriate.

4.2.1 Basic Concepts

Any valid analysis of observer performance must account for the fact that two fundamentally different kinds of errors can be made in a visual detection task: an observer can fail to detect an object feature when it is actually present ("false-negative error" or "miss"); or an object feature can be incorrectly "detected" when none, in fact, is present ("false-positive error" or "false alarm"). In the medical literature, this need is often met by reporting the performance of a diagnostic test in terms of its "sensitivity," the fraction of patients actually having a disease that is called "positive" by the test; and "specificity," the fraction of patients actually without the disease that is called "negative" (Lusted, 1978; Weinstein and Fineberg, 1980). This pair of indices distinguishes between the two kinds of error, but it suffers from an important limitation: The numerical values depend upon the "critical confidence level," or "decision criterion," that each observer adopts to distinguish "positive" image readings from "negative" readings (Metz, 1978; 1986a).

For example, consider the situation in which a radiologist reads each image in a collection of chest radiographs as "positive" or "negative" with regard to the presence of lung nodules. To avoid an unacceptably high number of false-positive readings, the radiologist presumably calls positive only those radiographs in which his confidence in the presence of a nodule exceeds some minimum acceptable level. Clearly, the sensitivity and specificity of the radiologist's readings could be calculated if the actual presence or absence of nodules in each radiograph were established subsequently by biopsy, clinical follow-up, etc.

Now suppose that the same radiologist reads the same radiographs more aggressively, in the sense that he requires less confidence in the presence of a nodule in order to issue a positive report. The sensitivity of the radiologist's readings will increase because some actually positive cases that had not previously exceeded the radiologist's "critical confidence level" will now correctly be called positive; but the specificity of the radiologist's readings will decrease because some of the marginally suspect cases previously called negative and now called positive will, in fact, be without nodules. Similarly, the radiologist's sensitivity would decrease, but his specificity would increase if he were to read the images more conservatively, issuing a positive report only if his confidence in the presence of a nodule were very high.

The radiologist's inherent ability to associate the appearance of an image with the likelihood that a lung nodule is actually present remains unchanged across these different sensitivities and specificities. Hence, the ability of a human observer to distinguish between two states of truth cannot be characterized by a single sensitivity-specificity pair. This problem can be overcome by determining all of the combinations of sensitivity and specificity that an imaging procedure provides in a particular detection task as the critical confidence level is varied over all possible settings, and by plotting one of these indices against the other in a unit square, as shown in Figure 4.1a. More commonly, TPF, which is equivalent to sensitivity, is plotted against FPF, which is equal to 1.0 minus specificity, thereby producing an ROC curve (Green and Swets, 1966; Metz, 1978; 1986a; Swets

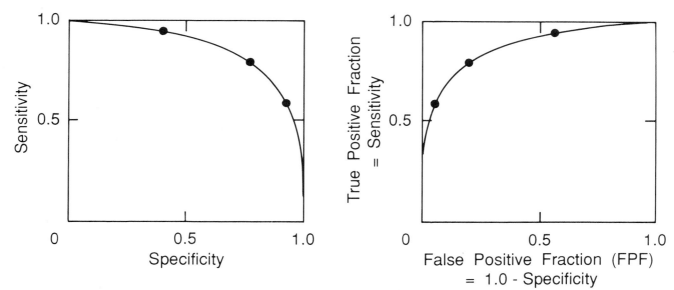

Fig. 4.1. (a) Examples of three possible combinations of sensitivity and specificity that can be obtained in image reading by the use of different settings of the critical confidence level (points) and the continuous trade off that is available between these quantities (curve). (b) The same combinations and relationship expressed in terms of TPF and FPF, the convention employed in ROC analysis.

and Pickett, 1982), as shown in Figure 4.1b. Receiver Operating Characteristic curves rise from the lower-left corner of the unit square; bend to the right with decreasing slope; and finally enter the upper-right corner of the square. High ROC curves represent better detection performance than low ones because with appropriate settings of the decision criterion, a larger TPF can be obtained on a higher ROC for any given FPF, or a smaller FPF can be obtained for a given true positive fraction. If ROC curves of interest do not intersect each other, detection performance can be summarized by the area under an ROC inside the unit square (Swets and Pickett, 1982; Metz, 1986a). Alternatively, ROCs can be compared in terms of the TPF values they provide at a particular FPF of practical interest (Swets and Pickett, 1982; McNeil and Hanley, 1984).

4.2.2 Receiver Operating Characteristic Curves from Confidence-Rating Data

Two different experimental approaches can be used to measure conventional ROC curves for imaging systems.

In the first approach, sometimes called the "Yes/No" method (Green and Swets, 1966), the observer views a series of images sequentially and is required to give a binary (*e.g.*, "positive" or "negative") response for each image. The series is then re-read on several occasions, with the reader motivated to use either a "stricter" or "more lenient" confidence threshold on each subsequent occasion. The observer's responses from each reading occasion can be compared with the truth about the cases and thus used to compute different {FPF, TPF} pairs, each of

which is plotted as a point in the unit square. Vertical and horizontal error bars can then be calculated for each point on the basis of binomial statistics (Green and Swets, 1966), and a smooth curve can be drawn near the points. This approach follows directly from the conceptual basis for ROC analysis, but it is experimentally inefficient, requiring each observer to read the series of images M times to generate estimates of M points on the Receiver Operating Characteristic curve.

The "rating method" is more efficient and is almost always used in practice. In this approach (Green and Swets, 1966; Goodenough *et al.*, 1974; Metz, 1979; Swets and Pickett, 1982), the observer is required to select one of several categories of confidence — usually represented by numerical ratings — to report his impression of the likelihood that each image arose from one or the other state of truth. These categories can be given qualitative labels such as: (1) definitely or almost definitely negative, (2) probably negative, (3) possibly positive, (4) probably positive and (5) definitely or almost definitely positive. It is not necessary for different observers to interpret these category labels in the same way; the essential requirement is that the labels provide an unambiguously ordered set of categories for each observer's relative confidence in the two states of truth. Also, for statistical efficiency, it is desirable that the category labels motivate the observer to generate combinations of FPF and TPF (as explained below) that are distributed more or less uniformly along the ROC curve. When the images included in an experiment are approximately half actually positive and half actually negative, this is accomplished if the observer uses the categories with roughly equal frequencies in responding to the combination of actually positive and actually negative images.

The idea that underlies the rating method is shown schematically in Figure 4.2. If the observer is asked to give a categorical rating to describe his confidence that each image is positive, then we can assume that he must set several boundaries on his continuous confidence scale and report the interval into which his impression of each image falls. To establish a five-category rating scale, *e.g.*, he would need to set four thresholds, or "category boundaries," like those shown in Figure 4.2. Suppose that the observer is required to use a five-category rating scale, such that a rating of 5 indicates the category of highest confidence in a positive diagnosis and 1 indicates the category of lowest confidence in a positive diagnosis. In other words, a rating of 1 represents the category of highest confidence in a negative diagnosis. In this situation, the cases that are rated as 5 can be interpreted by the data analyst as those that would be called "positive" in a "Yes/No" experiment for which the observer uses a very strict confidence threshold, and cases with any other rating can be interpreted as those that would be called "negative" in that experiment. From this viewpoint, the rating data yield a single combination of FPF and TPF — in other words, a single point on the ROC curve.

The same data can be considered in other ways, however. For example, the cases that were assigned a rating of 4 or 5 can be interpreted as those that would be called "positive" by the same observer in a "Yes/

No" experiment if he were using the less strict confidence threshold that corresponds to the boundary between Category 3 and Category 4 on the decision axis in Figure 4.2. Thus, the cases that are rated 4 or 5 can be scored as "positive" readings to produce a second point on the ROC curve, above and to the right of the first point. By proceeding in this way, the data analyst can calculate M-1 different points on an ROC curve from a single set of M-category rating data obtained in a single experiment. Usually five or six categories have been employed in confidence-rating experiments to obtain four or five points on the ROC curve in addition to points in the lower left and upper right corners of the unit square, through which we know a conventional ROC curve must pass. These numbers of categories represent a compromise between the desirability of obtaining as many ROC points as possible and the empirical fact that some observers find it difficult to partition subjective judgements into more than five or six categories. Recently, Rockette *et al.* (1992) suggested the use of a continuous confidence-judgement scale in ROC experiments to reduce the likelihood of "degenerate" data sets, which cause problems in curve fitting (Metz, 1989). They showed that the continuous and five-category scales gave equivalent results when data degeneracy was not problematic, and they found that the continuous scale was preferred by the radiologists who served as observers in their experiment.

Receiver Operating Characteristic curves are fitted

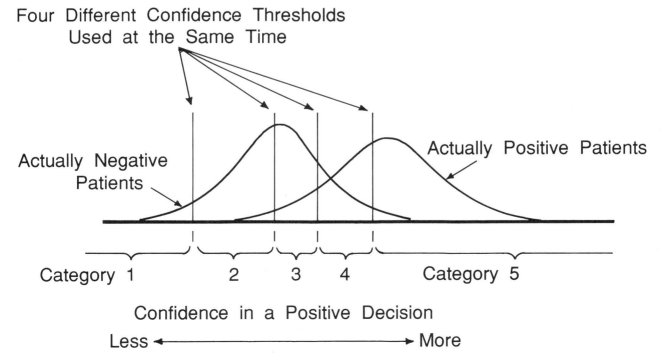

Fig. 4.2. The model upon which the "confidence-rating" method of measuring an ROC curve is based, sketched here for a five-category rating scale. To establish a rating scale with M discrete categories of confidence on the decision-variable axis, the observer must set M-1 different confidence thresholds simultaneously (from Metz, 1986a).

to confidence-rating data by maximum-likelihood estimation, using an assumption that the measured ROCs have the "binormal" form that plots as a straight line on "normal-deviate" axes (Swets, 1979; 1986; Swets and Pickett, 1982; Metz, 1986a). According to the binormal model, which includes two adjustable parameters, each ROC curve is assumed to have the same functional form as that implied by two "normal" (*i.e.*, Gaussian) decision-variable distributions with generally different means and standard deviations (Green and Swets, 1966; Swets, 1979; Egan, 1975). Empirically, this functional form has been found to provide satisfactory fits to ROC data generated in a very broad variety of situations (Swets, 1986). Conventional least-squares methods are not appropriate for fitting ROCs because the assumptions that underlie those methods are not valid for confidence-rating data (Metz, 1986b). Two approaches can be used when several sets of rating data (from repeated readings by the same or different observers) are available for estimation of a single ROC: The data sets can be fit individually and the resulting binormal curve parameters averaged, or the data can be pooled and then fit. The advantages and disadvantages of the two methods have been discussed by Metz (1986a).

A large and sometimes confusing variety of statistical tests is available for evaluating the statistical significance of differences between ROC curves. Most of these tests have been developed specifically for ROC analysis because most conventional statistical tests are not able to distinguish between differences in confidence-rating data that are due to changes in the ROC and differences that are due only to changes in the observer's use of the confidence-rating scale. The various tests apply to different experimental designs and address different null hypotheses. Statistical tests for differences between ROC curves have been reviewed by McNeil and Hanley (1984), Hanley (1989) and Metz (1986b; 1989). A new approach that employs "jackknifing" and analysis of variance was proposed recently by Dorfman *et al.* (1992).

4.2.3 Indices of Performance

4.2.3.1 The Area under the Receiver Operating Characteristic Curve (A$_z$) as an Index of Performance. An ROC curve represents all of the compromises between sensitivity and specificity that can be achieved by a diagnostic system as the confidence threshold is varied, and ROCs indicating better decision performance lie higher in the unit square. Therefore, the index A_z provides a summary of inherent discrimination performance that is independent of possible variations in the confidence threshold (Swets, 1979; Hanley and McNeil, 1982; Swets and Pickett, 1982). This area can be interpreted as the average value of sensitivity on the corresponding ROC if the system's specificity is selected randomly

between 0 and 1, or, equivalently, as the average value of specificity on the ROC if sensitivity is selected randomly between 0 and 1 (Metz, 1986a).

The univariate index A_z provides a useful basis for ranking imaging systems, and can be plotted as a function of any physical parameter of the imaging process (such as lesion size, spatial resolution or patient radiation exposure) to summarize the effect of that parameter on detectability. One must recognize that any univariate summary of detection performance can be misleading, however. For example, ROC curves having the same A_z value may provide substantially different sensitivities at a particular specificity of practical interest, or substantially different specificities at a selected sensitivity, because the two ROCs may cross inside the unit square. Similarly, an imaging system characterized by a lower A_z value may, in fact, provide better detection performance over a limited range of sensitivity or specificity than a system with a higher A_z value (Metz, 1989). Possibilities of this kind are inevitable with any univariate summary index because detection performance is described fully only by the complete ROC, which has at least two degrees of freedom.

4.2.3.2 Signal-to-Noise Ratio. An equivalent index of performance to A_z is d_a, defined as $\sqrt{2}$ times the standard normal deviate corresponding to the probability A_z; *i.e.*, $A_z = \phi(d_a/\sqrt{2})$, where ϕ represents the cumulative standard-normal distribution function. That is,

$$
\begin{aligned}
A_z &= \int_0^1 \text{TPF} \, d(\text{FPF}) \\
&= (2\pi)^{-1/2} \int_{-\infty}^{d_a/\sqrt{2}} e^{-z^2/2} \, dz.
\end{aligned}
\tag{4.1}
$$

Thus, the index d_a can be interpreted as an effective SNR and is a generalization of the index d', which applies only to binormal ROCs that are symmetric about the $-45°$ diagonal of the unit square (Simpson and Fitter, 1973; Swets, 1979). In effect, the value of d_a for a general ROC represents the d' value of a symmetric binormal ROC with the same area under it. It has, therefore, precisely the same normalization as the SNR_I, the Hotelling observer and the NPWMF discussed in Section 3 (*i.e.*, they use the average of the variances under the two hypotheses as the denominator of the SNR^2). If these SNRs are known, they can be used in place of d_a in Equation 4.1 to determine the area under the ROC curve when an ROC study is made using phantoms with the signal and noise characteristics discussed in Section 3.

4.3 Forced-Choice Analysis

Receiver Operating Characteristic analysis provides a more complete description of observer performance than other currently available techniques and, in principle, it can be applied to any two-alternative decision task. However, ROC experiments often require a substantial amount of time and effort by the observer, since each image reading must be graded on a confidence scale that the observer must attempt to hold constant during his participation in the experiment. In situations where only a summary index is sought and the full ROC is not required, "forced choice" methodology provides an alternative, and sometimes more efficient, approach.

4.3.1 Two-Alternative Forced-Choice Experiments

As noted in Section 4.2.3.1, the ROC area index A_z provides a useful summary of discrimination performance. Perhaps surprisingly, A_z can be measured directly in a "two-alternative forced-choice" (2-AFC) experiment (Green and Swets, 1966) without measurement of — or explicit reference to — the ROC curve.

The observer in a 2-AFC experiment views independent pairs of images together. One image in each pair is always actually positive, whereas the other is always actually negative, and the observer is required to state which image is positive (or negative). If the actually positive image is varied randomly in each pair (between left and right, say, with equal probability), then the percentage of correct decisions in this task can range from 0.5 (indicating chance performance) to 1 (indicating perfect performance). With this paradigm, the observer does not need to adopt any confidence threshold; instead, his impressions of the two images are compared with each other. It can be shown, under very general assumptions, that the expected fraction of correct decisions in this 2-AFC experiment equals the expected A_z that would be measured with the same images viewed one at a time in a conventional ROC experiment, (Green and Swets, 1966; Hanley and McNeil, 1982). Thus, if only the ROC area, A_z, is of interest, it can be measured directly by the 2-AFC paradigm, with some apparent saving in experimental effort.

The chief disadvantage of the 2-AFC approach lies in the fact that the trade-off between sensitivity and specificity (*i.e.*, the ROC curve) is never determined. Therefore, the result of a 2-AFC experiment cannot be used in a higher-order efficacy analysis involving costs and benefits (see Section 6.1.1), where a particular compromise between sensitivity and specificity must be considered. Although the 2-AFC paradigm can be more efficient than the ROC approach in terms of observer time, it is less efficient in terms of the number of images required for the experiment because greater statistical precision in the A_z index can be gained with a given number of images if confidence-rating data, which determine the ROC, are obtained from the observer (Hanley and McNeil, 1982). Thus, the 2-AFC technique should be considered for use primarily in situations where the A_z index provides an

adequate summary of performance and where observer time — rather than the number of images available with truth — is the scarce experimental resource.

4.3.2 Multiple-Alternative Forced-Choice Experiments

A generalization of the 2-AFC paradigm involves a task in which exactly one of $M > 2$ simultaneously-presented images (or locations in a single image) is actually positive, and the observer is required to identify the actually positive image (or location). The level of performance achieved by the observer is represented by the fraction of such trials in which his decision is correct (Green and Swets, 1966). For a given level of image quality, the difficulty of this "multiple-alternative forced-choice" (M-AFC) task increases with M, the number of images (or candidate locations) presented to the observer in each trial. The theoretical relationship among the probability of a correct response in an M-AFC trial, effective SNR and M is demonstrated in Table 4.1. Each SNR in Table 4.1 is equivalent to the d' value (Green and Swets, 1966) of an ROC curve that would be obtained if the multiple images (or image locations) used in each trial of the M-AFC experiment were interpreted individually in an ROC experiment.

An advantage of the M-AFC paradigm is that statistical power can be optimized, for any given level of image quality (SNR), by use of an appropriate value of M. The M-AFC technique also provides substantially better sampling statistics than 2-AFC experiments for a given number of decision trials and allows the investigation of observer performance at higher signal-to-noise ratios (Burgess, 1989).

It should be noted that the use of Elliot's tables (Table 4.1) involves an implicit, but rather strong assumption about the form of the ROC curve which would be obtained if the multiple images (or image locations) used in each trial of the M-AFC experiment were interpreted individually in an ROC experiment. This assumption is that the ROC would plot on "normal-deviate" axes (Green and Swets, 1966; Swets, 1979) as a straight line with unit slope, *i.e.*, that it would have the same form as an ROC arising from two Gaussian decision-variable distributions with

TABLE 4.1—*Signal-to-noise ratios theoretically required to achieve various probabilities of a correct response P (correct) in a forced-choice experiment involving M decision alternatives. Extracted from a more complete table by Elliot (1964)*

P (correct)	M = 8	M = 32	M = 256	M = 1,024
0.50	1.34	2.09	2.90	3.20
0.75	2.13	2.85	3.64	3.90
0.95	2.84	3.53	4.30	4.53
0.99	4.06	4.70	5.44	5.61

equal standard deviations. Any small departure from the strict validity of this assumption may not have a substantial effect on the inferred value of d' when M is small, but its impact will increase with M. Therefore, the M-AFC method with large numbers of decision alternatives must be used cautiously in observer-efficiency experiments.

Results of M-AFC experiments relevant to medical imaging have been reported by, *e.g.*, Burgess and Ghandeharian (1984a), Ishida *et al.* (1984) and Loo *et al.* (1984).

4.4 Test Patterns for Observer Performance Experiments

Both the ease with which observer performance experiments are conducted, and the results that those experiments provide, depend upon the objects about which decisions must be made and upon the images that are used as a basis for those decisions. Therefore, careful attention must be devoted to the selection of objects and images if the results of an observer performance experiment are to provide meaningful indicators of image quality. Several possible classes of objects and images are considered here.

4.4.1 Clinical Images

Questions of image quality in diagnostic medicine ultimately concern the ability of radiologists or other trained observers to correctly decide patients' states of health and disease from images made under clinical conditions. Therefore, observer performance experiments that employ clinical images can provide direct assessments of image quality, and such studies are preferred whenever they are feasible and scientifically valid. Several practical considerations often make the use of clinical images difficult, however.

In any objective evaluation of a diagnostic system, the true state of the object (*e.g.*, patient) from which each image is made must be known by the data analyst so that observers' responses can be compared with truth. Unfortunately, the establishment of diagnostic truth in clinical images is sometimes difficult, both in principle and in practice (because great effort may be required to determine the actual state of health or disease of a particular patient at a particular point in time "beyond a reasonable doubt"). Important issues that must be confronted in establishing truth in clinical evaluation studies have been reviewed elsewhere (Ransohoff and Feinstein, 1978; Swets and Pickett, 1982; Metz, 1986a; Begg and McNeil, 1988). Particular attention must be focused on biases that may be caused by the omission of clinical cases for which truth is particularly difficult to establish (Ransohoff and Feinstein, 1978; Gray *et al.*, 1984).

The detectability of a lesion in an image obviously depends not only upon the physical properties of the imaging system, but also upon the size, contrast, etc. of the lesion in question and upon the characteristics of non-lesion structures and other lesions that are (or may be) present in the images. More generally, the ability of an observer to discriminate visually between two classes of objects or "cases" depends upon the subtlety of the differences between the two classes in question. Therefore, the result of an observer-performance experiment obtained with a particular set of images — and so, according to an operational definition of image quality, the quality of those images — depends not only upon the physical properties of the images, such as spatial resolution and noise level, but also upon the characteristics of the particular actually positive cases (patients) and actually negative cases from which the images were made. This dependence is inconvenient, but it is consistent with the common observation that different imaging systems can excel in depicting different classes of scenes and in different image-based tasks. Similarly, image quality as defined here depends upon the skill of the observer who reads the images, but this dependence also is appropriate because different imaging systems may be best when used by observers with different training or experience. Ideally, all observers who perform a particular image-reading task would possess the highest level of skill that is humanly attainable; in reality, however, images are read by observers with diverse skills.

Because the results of an image-evaluation study generally depend upon the cases and observers that the study employs, care must be taken to ensure that those cases and observers are selected appropriately. It is important to recognize that sampling issues must be addressed in any evaluation study, and that ROC methodology is no more demanding in this regard than other methods of analysis that provide less meaningful descriptions of detection performance (Metz, 1986a).

In designing a visual-detection experiment for the evaluation of image quality, one must decide first whether an absolute measure of the detectability of some class of diagnostic features or some particular disease is desired, or whether the goal is more simply to rank alternative imaging procedures (Metz, 1989). The sampling issues that must be confronted in these two kinds of experiments can be quite different.

Reliable absolute measurements of disease detectability in a defined patient population are often extremely difficult to obtain — in part because the sample of patients included in the study must accurately reflect the population of patients at large about which conclusions are to be drawn — and many sources of potential bias must be taken into account (Begg and McNeil, 1988). For example, an experiment that attempts to measure the absolute detectability of lung nodules by chest radiography must ensure that the distribution of nodule sizes is the same in the study sample as in the defined population of interest because the detectability of a nodule depends on its size. Formal "stratified sampling" techniques (Kendall and Stuart, 1976) have not yet been used formally in medical imaging, but may prove useful for reliable absolute measurements of system performance. In the detection of lung nodules, for example, these techniques can help to ensure that an appropriate distribution of nodule sizes is used in a study (Metz, 1988).

The absolute detectability obtained in medical imaging depends not only on the difficulty of the cases, but also on the experience and skill of the observers (*e.g.*, radiologists) who read the images: Experienced mammographers have been shown to perform better than general radiologists in using xeromammograms to discriminate between malignant and benign breast lesions (Getty *et al.*, 1988), for example. Therefore, if reliable absolute measurements of detectability are to be obtained from a medical imaging study, the relevant population of observers must be defined, and the sample of observers employed in the study must accurately represent that population. Similarly, to measure accurately the absolute detectability of disease that would be obtained in routine clinical practice, the conditions under which images are read in the study, *e.g.*, reading time, ambient light level, etc., must represent those that would be used in clinical practice.

Studies that seek only to rank systems are often much more straightforward. Sampling considerations still require attention in the study design, but now the only requirement is that these factors do not affect the ranking of the systems; their effects on absolute detectability are no longer of primary concern. The key need becomes one of ensuring that a system which would provide superior diagnostic performance in its real-world application is found better in the study, and that two systems providing equivalent performance in the real world are found equivalent by the study. Issues that should be addressed in selecting clinical cases for an observer performance study that seeks to rank imaging systems have been discussed by Metz (1988; 1989).

Carefully designed clinical image-evaluation studies can be done, and useful conclusions can be drawn from them (see, *e.g.*, Swets and Pickett, 1982; Metz, 1986a), but studies that use non-clinical images — though subject to other limitations, noted below — are less demanding and often adequate.

4.4.2 Phantom Images

Some of the practical difficulties of clinical images in observer performance experiments are overcome by the use of specially-designed inanimate objects ("phantoms") instead of human patients. "Truth" is

defined by the phantom's construction, and the features to be detected or distinguished by the observers are readily controlled. Images of carefully designed phantoms can accurately represent virtually all of the physical aspects of the clinical image-forming process. The task of selecting object features and/or images with an appropriate level of difficulty has been discussed by Metz (1989).

The chief limitation of phantom images in observer performance experiments usually is the problem of designing and manufacturing phantoms that represent clinical object structures with realism sufficient to ensure that the experiment's results are similar to those that would be obtained in clinical practice. Accurate representation of complex anatomical background is often difficult or impossible, particularly because that background must vary from image to image if it is to represent the normal anatomical variation among patients which typically complicates clinical image interpretation. Generation of large numbers of phantom images sometimes can be laborious, especially when the positioning and/or background of the phantom is varied in a controlled way to simulate clinical conditions.

Phantom images are most useful in observer performance studies when the determination of truth in clinical cases is difficult and an absence of realistic, variable background structure is considered unlikely to affect the results sought from the study.

4.4.3 Computer-Generated Images

Large numbers of images for use in an observer performance study can be generated quickly and inexpensively by digital computer and subsequently displayed on film or a video monitor. Knowledge of the physical processes associated with a particular imaging modality often can be used to produce images that closely approximate those that could be obtained more laboriously with phantoms. Object features to be detected and/or background structures can be varied stochastically with relative ease. A unique advantage of computer-generated images in research is their ability to simulate the images that would be produced by hypothetical imaging modalities or by various combinations of imaging parameters in existing modalities.

The chief disadvantage of computer-generated images is that the accuracy with which they represent real images is sometimes limited or unknown, either because inclusion of the full complexity of the physical image-forming process may be difficult or because computer-modelled object features and background structures may be oversimplified.

4.4.4 Hybrid Images

In an attempt to combine the advantages of clinical and computer-simulated images in observer performance experiments that involve lesion detection, actually normal clinical images can be modified by computer to represent the inclusion of abnormal object features. Hybrid images of this kind reduce the difficulty of determining clinical truth; allow a detection experiment to include lesions with any desired size, shape and contrast; and automatically include realistic — indeed, real — variations in normal anatomical background.

Hybrid images are produced most easily with modalities such as CT and scintigraphy, in which clinical images are readily available in digital form and the imaging process is essentially linear, but they can be generated also in other modalities such as screen/film radiography by digitization of analog images and appropriate attention to sensitometric effects. Simulated lesions superimposed upon actually normal clinical images must take into account the spatial resolution of the imaging system and must include the effects of any (significant) perturbations which the presence of a lesion would impose on the detected radiation field.

4.5 Summary

Image quality in medicine must be judged in terms of the extent to which a class of images allows real observers, such as radiologists, to decide correctly each patient's state of health or disease. Image quality in this sense can be assessed experimentally.

Receiver Operating Characteristic analysis, which estimates all of the combinations of "sensitivity" and "specificity" available from a diagnostic imaging procedure, provides the most complete description of observer performance and, thus, of image quality. Experiments based on the forced-choice paradigm can be more efficient than those which use ROC analysis when images with known truth are readily available, but their results cannot be used in higher-order efficacy analyses. Other approaches to the evaluation of visual detection performance, such as the method of constant stimulus and "contrast-detail" measurements (see Section 2), are substantially less reliable and cannot be recommended broadly.

Questions of image quality in diagnostic medicine ultimately concern the ability of radiologists or other trained observers to correctly decide patients' states of health and disease from images made under clinical conditions. Therefore, observer performance experiments that employ clinical images can provide direct assessments of image quality, and such studies are recommended whenever they are feasible and scientifically valid. Practical considerations often make the use of clinical images difficult, however. Alternative approaches include the use of real images of inanimate objects ("phantoms"), wholly synthetic images generated by computer, or hybrid images in which simulated abnormalities are added digitally to actually-normal clinical images. Each of these alternatives provides a different compromise between realism and convenience.

MTF, and W_n, the noise power spectrum. The first two factors define the scaling relationship between the object and image. Usually, a calibration phantom is used to generate the scaling relationship and measurements are made under conditions comparable to the intended conditions of use of the imaging system.

The kinds of physical signals generated from objects, phantoms or patients are discussed in Appendix A. Where possible, one attempts to define these signals in such a way that they are intrinsic properties of the object and independent of the imaging conditions. Frequently this can be done by, for example, defining the relative activity of neighboring materials or tissues in the nuclear medicine case, or by working with the logarithm of the detected signal, *i.e.*, optical density, in radiography. This independence is not always possible, however; in MRI the relative signal strengths depend upon several time-scales characteristic of the imaging technique. The calibration technique should control for such parameters; *i.e.*, they should be specifiable and repeatable.

A critical ingredient of such a calibration technique is the phantom itself. Much experience has been gained in recent years indicating that the physical properties of some phantom materials may change over time. This problem must be addressed, either through the design of a stable calibration phantom, or a stable calibration transfer technique, in order to achieve consensus measurement methodology.

5.3.4.1 Calculation of Signal-to-Noise Ratio. For the simple detection or discrimination task, the SNR_I is given by combining the NEQ with a function $\Delta \bar{f}(\nu)$, representing the task to be performed (see Sections 3.3 and 3.4):

$$ SNR_I^2 = K^2 \int \frac{|\Delta \bar{f}(\nu)|^2 MTF^2(\nu)}{W_n(\nu)} \, d\nu. \qquad (5.3) $$

Models for predicting the SNR for other tasks are available, but may be of daunting complexity. One approach is to assume (see also, Hanson, 1983) that they take the form

$$ \frac{\nu^{2n} K^2 MTF^2(\nu)}{W_n(\nu)}, \qquad (5.4) $$

where the choice of the value for n depends upon the specific task.

5.3.4.2 Advantages and Disadvantages. The ideal observer approach has two main advantages. Firstly, it allows one to predict the best possible performance that the imaging system could achieve for a specific task. Secondly, being analytical, it allows one to determine rapidly how changes in various parameters associated with the imaging system will affect its performance. However, the drawbacks of this approach are, firstly, that, at present, an optimal performance is only predictable for a very limited number of simple situations. Eventually it may be possible to extend it to a greater range of tasks and imaging problems. Secondly, the difficulty in making measurements of system parameters, such as MTF and Weiner spectrum, should not be underestimated. While the basic steps in this process have been outlined above, in practice, achieving accurate measurements is not a trivial task. Thirdly, the relationship between the results of the ideal observer approach and the result of clinical evaluation is unknown at present.

5.4 Quality of the Displayed Data

The application of signal detection theory to the real observer allows us to measure directly the actual performance achieved in a specific imaging situation.

Two approaches are available, one being to use the rating paradigm to generate the ROC curve, the other to use the forced choice approach. These techniques are discussed in detail in Sections 4.2.2 and 4.3.1, respectively. A number of parameters can be generated from the data, including A_z and d_a, the latter measuring the SNR achieved by the real observer. It should be noted that, in both cases, it is necessary to train the observers in the task they are to perform so that the results are not influenced by the effect of learning.

5.4.1 Rating Technique

The relationship between the number of images, as well as the relative number of normal and abnormal images, and statistical power is very complicated, but various aspects of this subject are discussed in Hanley and McNeil (1982; 1983), McNeil and Hanley (1984), Metz *et al.* (1984), Metz (1989) and Swets and Pickett (1982). The number of images needed in an ROC (or forced choice) experiment can vary widely, depending strongly upon both the magnitude of the difference in detectability that actually exists — or is considered negligible — and the extent to which ROC estimates are correlated across imaging conditions and/or observers (Swets and Pickett, 1982). These factors should be estimated in a pilot study.

For each image, the observer is asked to grade his/her confidence in the degree of normality/abnormality. Either a discrete five-point scale, such as that described in Section 4.2.2, or a continuous "subjective probability" scale can be employed (Rockette *et al.*, 1992).

The cumulative total of responses for each rating category is calculated; this will give pairs of true and false positive response rates from which the ROC curve can be plotted. For example, the five rating categories will yield four points on the ROC curve.

Curve fitting and index calculation can be performed using the programs devised by Metz (1989).

5.4.2 Forced Choice Technique

Each presentation consists of a group of images, one of which is abnormal and the others normal. The position of the abnormal image is varied randomly among presentations.

As this approach assumes that the observer is aware of the signal parameter information, a reference copy of the signal should be placed in the image outside the normal field. It is also assumed that the observer is aware of the possible signal location within each image, so it is important to provide location markers to indicate the precise location at which the signal may appear.

The observer is asked to identify the abnormal image in each group.

The value of d' or d_a corresponding to the observer's proportion of correct choices is then found from the tables published by Elliot (1964), with due attention paid to the caveat noted in Section 4.3.2. This value can then be converted to the ROC area index A_z if that is desired, by use of the formula $A_z = \phi(d_a/\sqrt{2})$, where $\phi(-)$ represents the cumulative standard-normal distribution function.

To achieve acceptably small sampling errors (*e.g.*, less than five percent), typically, 200 to 400 trials are required.

5.4.3 Comparison of Rating and Forced-Choice Techniques

In order to achieve a given degree of accuracy, the forced-choice technique is less demanding of observer time, but requires more images. Also, it only allows one to predict the summary measures of the ROC curve and not the curve itself. Choice of technique will thus depend upon the particular situation but, in general, the rating technique appears the best for clinical images and the forced choice approach when using synthetic data.

5.5 Relative Role of the Ideal and Real Observers in Measuring Quality

The SNR_I provides the measure of the upper limit of the performance achievable by any observer. This approach also allows a rapid assessment to be made of the effect of altering imaging parameters on signal-to-noise ratio. However, there are a number of limitations to its application as a general measure of image quality which must be addressed.

The real observer allows one to measure the performance on real clinical patient data, under clinical conditions and is, at present, the most realistic measure of performance. However, it is not practicable to use the real observer as the primary assessment of image quality as the technique is unduly time consuming. Its main limitation is that it only provides a measure of SNR at one specific point out of a whole range of various operating conditions. For example, to measure the effect of changing a parameter, such as exposure time, a new experiment must be done.

5.6 Suggested Approach to Measuring Image Quality Parameters

Based on the ideas presented in Sections 3 and 4, it is suggested that image quality could be assessed in the following way. However, it should be emphasized that variations on this approach may prove to be necessary in the light of experience with different imaging modalities.

5.6.1 Experimental Procedure

It is suggested that the following steps be employed for the experimental determination of quality.

Firstly, the clinical problem, or group of problems, for which the imaging technique(s) is to be applied should be defined. This problem may then need to be redefined, if possible, as a discrimination task with a finite number of known outcomes. This having been done, it is possible to design the test pattern set.

A variety of parameters should be measured in order to define the performance of the imaging equipment; these should include the MTF, K and Wiener spectrum of the system. All measurements should be made under the conditions that are applicable to the imaging test. If it proves possible to obtain all these measures, the NEQ can be calculated.

If the test pattern and task permit, the SNR_I should be calculated for the appropriate range(s) of operating conditions. If, however, the ideal observer approach is not practicable, then an approximate model should be tried.

Based on the measurements of the ideal or quasi-ideal SNRs, the operating conditions, corresponding to the maximum SNR, should be chosen. If, however, the SNRs cannot be calculated, the relevant operating conditions may need to be determined using one of the test patterns described in Section 2.3.

Using the same (or similar) test image set to that above, measure the ROC curves for the chosen operating conditions. From these ROC curves, the SNR_R can be calculated.

5.6.2 Use of Image Quality Parameters

The MTF, K, NPS and NEQ all provide measures of the performance of the imaging device. Noise equivalent quanta has the advantage of combining the three other parameters and it may prove to be of great value in assessing equipment performance.

From the measurements outlined above, it is possible to derive performance indices, SNR_R and, in certain cases, SNR_I (or the SNR of a quasi-ideal observer). These SNRs provide the most comprehensive measures of image quality, but their relative value depends upon the reason why quality is being measured. In the context of the clinical task, four questions are relevant:

1. Does imaging modality X perform better than modality Y?
2. Is instrument A better than B for carrying out the task, both instruments being of the same modality?
3. How does varying the instrument's parameters alter its ability to carry out the task?
4. What is the best performance that the instrument can actually achieve?

The use of SNR can give a measure which is independent of the modality. This allows instruments of either the same or different modalities to be compared. This permits problems (1) and (2) to be addressed, although in answering question (1) cognizance must be taken of the effect of the physical, chemical and physiological properties of the lesions and surrounding tissues on image contrast when using different imaging techniques. While the comparison can be made using either SNR_I or SNR_R, there are potential limitations. It should be remembered that many types of task do not permit SNR_I to be calculated. Also, since SNR_R represents the performance achieved under the particular conditions of data presentation chosen for the experiment, changes in data display may significantly alter the signal-to-noise ratio.

Signal-to-noise ratio of the real observer is the performance achieved by the real observer. A comparison with SNR_I measures how closely the actual performance approaches to the ideal and, therefore, whether there are any further improvements to be gained by modifying data presentation, *e.g.*, image reconstruction algorithms, data processing and image display. This allows question (3) to be investigated. Such a comparison is possible if, and only if, the SNR can be determined for both ideal and real observers for the same objects, which may not necessarily be lesions in clinical images.

A plot of SNR_I as a function of operating condition shows the best achievable performance of the device, bearing in mind the very specific conditions under which SNR_I can be calculated. Thus, in these circumstances, question (4) can be readily answered. However, as has been emphasized several times, there may be many situations which cannot be modelled in a way that will allow the calculation of the signal-to-noise ratio of the ideal observer.

Finally, it is important to consider whether the measured differences in the quality of images are relevant. The difference must be significant in terms of the clinical task. For example, system A may detect smaller lesions than system B, but if clinical symptoms do not develop until the lesion has at least reached the size detectable by system B, then the measured difference may be clinically irrelevant. Therefore, serious consideration must be given to the need to specify the level of quality which is to be regarded as clinically useful.

It should be emphasized that even in circumstances where only the ROC measurements of SNR_R are reported, it is essential that physical measurements necessary to characterize the imaging system used are given. Such measurements facilitate the understanding of the physical conditions needed to obtain the study's results in clinical practice, and serve to define the state-of-art of the modality studied.

6. Future Work

6.1 Image Quality in the Diagnostic Process

In this Report, methods have been outlined by which the quality of the data produced by clinical imaging systems can be judged. The approach starts with the definition of a task and finishes with measures of quality in terms of the efficiency with which the particular imaging technique allows this task to be accomplished. This efficiency is measured in two steps. The first is in terms of what can be achieved with the acquired data using a statistical analysis which may, in certain circumstances, provide a measure of the best possible performance. The second step measures the performance of the task by observers using the displayed data. Thus, it is possible to compare the actual performance with the "best" achievable. This is not intended to be the definitive approach to measuring quality and will need to be modified in the light of experience gained in applying it to specific imaging modalities.

If the proposed approach is to be of value, then it must meet two criteria. Firstly, can the results of the quality assessment be used to indicate what contribution the image data is making towards a clinical diagnosis which will influence the management of the patient? It is not sufficient to simply measure how good the device is at carrying out what may, in some circumstances, be a very limited task. Secondly, can the proposed method of quality assessment be applied to a range of different types of imaging devices?

6.1.1 Image Quality and Clinical Diagnosis

The six-level model of efficacy was introduced in Section 1.5. The work in this Report bridges the gap between levels 1 and 2; measures of technical efficacy, such as transfer functions and levels of noise power, have been related to diagnostic accuracy. But it is also necessary to demonstrate that the approach provides information which can be used to study efficacy at higher levels.

The effectiveness of the quality measure is largely determined by the chosen task. While the use of the ideal observer to assess the quality of the acquired data in terms of classification tasks is relatively well understood, the application to the problem of estimation is much less clear. However, as described in Section 3.9, there would appear to be a framework encompassing the two. The clinical applicability of the quality measure depends on the extent to which the information relevant to a particular clinical task can be identified in terms of such classification tasks. The formulation of clinical tasks in these simple terms is a problem which has not been given much thought but one whose resolution is overdue.

Because of the need for simple tasks, quality assessment using the approaches outlined in Section 3 cannot, at present, utilize real clinical data. However, the assessment of the displayed image can be done using real clinical data. The ROC curve allows one to measure the trade-off between true-positive and false-positive response rates. Looked at in terms of clinical parameters, it allows measurement of the sensitivity and specificity of the imaging technique.

In performing a diagnostic procedure, one pays a price (in terms of money and the risk of possible complications) to gain information that may be beneficial in subsequent patient management. The "information" that is gained regarding the actual state of health or disease can be measured and described, in a statistical sense, with ROC methodology.

Cost-benefit analysis can be used to relate the results of an ROC analysis to higher-order efficacy analyses in which the benefits and costs of true-positive, true-negative, false-positive and false-negative decisions are taken into account.

Although an ROC curve describes all of the trade-offs that can be realized among the relative frequencies of true-positive, false-negative, true-negative and false-positive diagnostic decisions, the particular compromise that is most efficacious depends both upon the prevalence of the disease in question in the population studied and upon the "utilities" or "values," i.e., the benefits and costs, of the various kinds of correct and incorrect decisions in a particular diagnostic setting. The optimal compromise among the relative frequencies of the various kinds of decisions, i.e., the optimal "operating point" on the ROC, can be studied in terms of the "expected value" or "expected net benefit" of a diagnostic system when the system is applied to a particular population of patients (McNeil et al., 1975; Metz et al., 1975; Metz, 1978; Swets and Swets, 1979; Swets and Pickett, 1982; Sainfort, 1991). In effect, the benefits and costs of each kind of decision are combined with the prevalence of the disease in question to find the combination of TPF and FPF on an ROC that yields the highest benefit, on the average. One can then compare this maximum benefit of the decisions with the "overhead cost" of doing the diagnostic procedure to determine its "expected net benefit." The components of benefit and cost that should be taken into account depend on the level of efficacy considered and may require measurements of subjective utilities (Keeny and Raiffa, 1976; Edwards, 1977). General issues that arise when higher-level efficacy analyses are approached in terms of ROC analysis have been reviewed by Swets and Pickett (1982).

6.1.2 Applicability to Other Imaging Devices

As stated in Section 3, the techniques for assessing the quality of the acquired data are most readily applicable to systems which are linear, or at least linearizable over the range of operating conditions, and shift invariant. Where the latter condition is not met, results indicating the average performance can be calculated. It is not envisaged that these conditions will prove to be a major limitation in practice and further work is being carried out by the ICRU to apply this approach to other devices. Some very general comments on the problems likely to be encountered with various imaging modalities are to be found in Appendix A.

To assess the performance in terms of acquired data, it is necessary to make measurements in terms of signals which represent intrinsic properties of the object and are independent of imaging conditions.

While, as pointed out in Section 3.2, this poses few problems for many imaging techniques, *e.g.*, in radiology the relationship between x-ray quanta and film density is well understood, certain modalities may pose problems, in particular in MRI where the basic information is dependent upon the time sequence of signals.

6.2 Conclusions

The proposed method provides an approach to assessing image quality which is sufficiently open ended to allow it to be applied to wider questions of diagnostic efficacy, yet sufficiently general to encompass most, if not all, types of imaging systems. However, it must be emphasized that the measurement of the various system parameters is not a trivial task and further detailed work is required.

Appendix A

Medical Imaging Devices

This Appendix gives a short overview of the most commonly encountered medical imaging modalities. In particular, the factors affecting the performance of the techniques are highlighted. The applicability to each modality of the proposed approach for measuring image quality is discussed, albeit only briefly, as it is intended that this will be the subject of future reports.

A.1 X-Ray

A.1.1 Planar Projection Imaging

A.1.1.1 Basic Imaging Technique. The attenuating properties of body tissues to x-ray photons of the range used in diagnostic radiology is determined principally by the photo-electric effect and Compton scattering. In a typical x-ray imaging system, photons emitted by an x-ray tube enter the patient where they may be absorbed, transmitted without interaction, or scattered. An image is formed from the emergent photons by their interaction with a suitable detector. Many different types of image receptor are used in diagnostic imaging systems (*e.g.*, x-ray film, fluorescent screens for cassette recording and image intensifiers) and all form an image by the absorption of energy from the photon flux leaving the patient. This image consists of a two-dimensional projection of the attenuating properties of all the tissues in the three-dimensional volume along the path of the x rays. The imaging photons are either primary photons which have passed through the patient without interacting, or secondary photons which derive from an interaction within the patient. The former contribute useful information to the image regarding internal structure, while the latter carry little information and merely contribute to the background signal which degrades contrast and signal-to-noise ratio.

The spatial resolution in planar projection imaging is of the order of 0.1 to 0.5 mm, the sharpness of the image depending upon the size of the focal spot (Doi, 1965) and the blurring introduced by the detector. The latter effect is discussed for screen film systems by, *e.g.*, Fisher (1982) and in ICRU Report 41 (ICRU, 1986).

The image noise, the radiographic mottle, is a result of both photon emission and reception being statistical processes. In addition, there are contributions from spatial fluctuations in the number of x-ray quanta absorbed in the intensifying screens caused by inhomogeneities in the phosphor coating (the structure mottle) and spatial non-uniformities in film sensitivity resulting from variations in the number of silver halide grains per unit area (film granularity) (Barnes, 1982). The major contribution to noise is quantum mottle, although at very low and very high optical densities and very high spatial frequencies, film granularity dominates.

A.1.1.2 Applicability of the Proposed Technique for Measuring Image Quality. The technique for measuring image quality is well-suited to planar x-ray imaging. The conversion of the analog image data to a numerical form requires careful calibration, in particular to standardize the effect of film response on image contrast. The measurement of the quality of the acquired data is considered further in Section D.2, while assessment of the quality of displayed data is described by Metz (1986a), for example.

A.1.2 Digital X-Ray Imaging

A.1.2.1 Basic Imaging Technique. Conventional radiological imaging systems record and display data in analog form. This analog image can be digitized using a scanning laser microdensitometer (Schwenker and Eger, 1985). There are advantages if the need to use film can be completely avoided. By means of an analog-to-digital converter, the image on an intensifier, stimulated luminescence plate or ionographic chamber can be converted directly into a digital format. Alternatively, a digital image can be created by scanning an x-ray beam with a slit collimator and an associated receptor system (such as, a bank of solid state detectors) across a region of the patient in so-called scanned projection radiography. The digital image can be stored on magnetic media or on optical disc, and can be interfaced with a film imaging system to make a permanent copy of an image.

Digital radiographic systems have several advantages. The image can be interrogated over the full range of pixel values in the data set by appropriate windowing; the digital image can be manipulated in several ways to improve perceptibility of image features; and image storage and retrieval are facilitated.

The digitization of the x-ray image often results in some loss of spatial resolution compared with the analog image. The extent to which resolution is compromised depends upon the technique employed. For example, analog film must be digitized to at least $2,048 \times 2,048$ pixels to give chest radiographs of comparable quality to analog images (MacMahon *et al.*, 1986), while digital fluorographic systems require

TV cameras capable of between 1,000 and 2,000 lines to give acceptable image reproduction.

In addition to the quantum noise encountered in planar imaging, noise will also be introduced into digital radiographic systems from various electronic sources. For example, in digital fluorographic systems there is TV camera noise, structure noise in the intensifier or photostimulable phosphor, and quantization noise from the analog-to-digital converters (Arnold and Scheibe, 1984; Harrison and Kotre, 1986).

A.1.2.2 Applicability of the Proposed Technique for Measuring Image Quality. Digital x-ray imaging lends itself to the methods of measuring performance recommended in this Report. Particular consideration needs to be given, however, to the effects of image digitization on image quality; see, for example, Giger and Doi (1985; 1987).

A.1.3 Computed Tomographic Imaging

A.1.3.1 Basic Imaging Technique. X-ray CT uses the same principle as analog and digital planar projection x-ray imaging, *i.e.*, an x-ray tube that projects an x-ray beam through the body, and some form of radiation detector to measure the intensity of the transmitted beam. The x-ray beam is collimated to a fan-shape that passes through a transverse section, or "slice," of the body. The detector system is a bank of individual scintillation or gas ionization detectors arranged in the same plane as the fan-beam, such that the beam, after emerging from the body, strikes the bank of detectors. The signal generated is proportional to the intensity of the transmitted x-ray beam and, hence, the negative of its logarithm is linearly proportional to the total attenuation along the path connecting the x-ray tube with the detector. A scan consists of moving the x-ray source (and sometimes also the detectors) in a plane so that the beam enters the body at a variety of angles over a range of at least 180°, and preferably 360°. In this way, attenuation data for many ray-paths at different angles and at different spatial offsets are obtained.

The signals from each detector are digitized, with each sample representing an intensity measurement for a different beam angle. Some preprocessing is performed on the data, such as taking the logarithm (so as to obtain a measure of attenuation, rather than intensity) and performing corrections for various distortions (such as detector non-linearity). A CT image of the body slice is then reconstructed from the data by a digital computer. The reconstruction algorithm is based on the filtered backprojection of the detected ray-sums. The physical quantity is attenuation coefficient, and the intensity of each picture element (pixel) of the image therefore represents the x-ray attenuation coefficient at the corresponding location in the body.

Spatial resolution in the image plane is determined by the dimensions of the detector apertures and any other collimators that may be present, and also by the sampling intervals. In general, the sampling rate is high enough so that this is not a limitation. Spatial resolution in the direction perpendicular to the image, or slice width, is determined by the collimator dimensions in that direction. Image noise, in a well-designed system, is limited by the number of detected x-ray quanta within the sampling interval, although the noise spectrum is altered by the image reconstruction algorithm.

Artifacts are an important consideration in x-ray CT, one example being the "beam-hardening" artifact. Since the attenuation coefficient is a function of effective beam energy, the attenuation caused by a given tissue location depends on the energy, or "hardness," of the x-ray beam at this point. This, in turn, depends on how much tissue the beam has already passed through and, hence, varies from ray to ray. This results in a distortion of intensity values, particularly around bony regions. Various corrections have been developed for such artifacts.

A.1.3.2 Applicability of the Proposed Technique for Measuring Image Quality. The proposed technique is readily applicable to CT imaging, although consideration needs to be given to the problems of artifacts, such as those created by bony regions, and to the dependence of image quality upon the details of the image-reconstruction algorithm that is employed. This particular application is discussed in Section D.4.

A.2 Nuclear Medicine

A.2.1 Planar Projection Imaging

A.2.1.1 Basic Imaging Technique. In nuclear medicine, images are produced showing the *in vivo* distribution of a pharmaceutical by labelling it with a radionuclide and detecting the gamma radiation as it emerges from the body. The imaging is performed with a gamma-camera which consists of a large scintillation crystal, some 40 to 50 cm in diameter, viewed by an array of photomultiplier tubes. By processing the signals from the photomultipliers, a pair of electronic signals representing the x and y spatial coordinates of the scintillation produced by the gamma-ray can be calculated. This is then used either to produce an analog image on a cathode ray tube (CRT) display or a digital image for computer processing (Sharp *et al.*, 1985).

The formation of an image in the crystal depends upon the use of a lead collimator having several thousand parallel holes running through it. This limits the gamma-radiation hitting the crystal to that travelling in a direction parallel to the axes of the holes, all obliquely incident radiation being absorbed by the lead. Imaging is thus achieved by excluding a large proportion of the radiation emitted from the patient, rather than by focusing it as in conventional photography. This is the principal cause of the low photon density found in these images.

As with x rays, the radiation will be absorbed and scattered in its passage through tissue to the detector. While it is crucial to the image formation process in transmission imaging, absorption will degrade quality in emission imaging.

Given a target tissue with a particular radiopharmaceutical concentration at a given point and adjacent tissue in which the concentration is different, the contrast between the two is given by a complex function which involves concentration, tissue thickness, the linear attenuation coefficient of each intervening tissue and the amount of scattered radiation detected.

In planar nuclear medicine imaging, resolution depends upon the dimensions of the holes in the collimator and the accuracy with which the position of the detected gamma-ray in the scintillation crystal can be calculated, the intrinsic resolution. The Compton scattering of radiation in the patient, prior to detection by the camera, also degrades resolution. Spatial resolution deteriorates with increasing distance from the collimator face but, for the parallel hole collimator, does not vary across the field of view. Typically the resolution is 5 mm full-width at half-maximum height on the collimator face, increasing to 1 cm at 10 cm from the collimator. Random noise is described by Poisson statistics, but variations in gamma camera uniformity may add a non-stochastic component.

A.2.1.2 Applicability of the Proposed Technique for Measuring Image Quality. The application of the technique for measuring image quality to planar projection imaging is discussed in Section D.2. In practice, care must be taken in calculating quality of the acquired data as the gamma camera system is not spatially invariant owing to non-uniformities in the camera response and, also, the MTF is dependent on distance from the collimator. The proposal for assessing the quality of the displayed data is well-suited to radionuclide images, and its use has already been reported by several groups, *e.g.*, Houston *et al.* (1979).

A.2.2 Single Photon Emission Computed Tomography

A.2.2.1 Basic Imaging Technique. Tomographic images are most commonly produced by taking a series of images as the gamma-camera (see Section A.2.1.1) is rotated around the patient (Gemmell, 1989), although specialized detectors have been constructed to improve the balance between spatial resolution and sensitivity (Evans *et al.*, 1986; Stod-

dart and Stoddart, 1979). The tomographic image is then reconstructed by "back-projecting" the image data obtained at each angle after first filtering to reduce artifacts (Gemmell, 1989). This reconstruction process results in image noise being "colored," *i.e.*, containing spatial structure, and with a texture that varies radially across the image.

The spatial resolution achieved in the single photon emission computed tomography (SPECT) is somewhat worse than in planar imaging, primarily due to the effect of data sampling and the cut-off frequency associated with the reconstruction filter; the loss in resolution at the center of rotation typically is some 10 to 30 percent greater than the planar value. One advantage of tomography is that resolution does not vary so markedly with distance from the detectors as in planar imaging, although this means that the resolution close to the detectors is similar to that at the center of rotation, *i.e.*, some 10 to 30 percent worse than the corresponding planar resolution 20 cm from the collimator (Larsson, 1980).

As the effect of tomography is to reduce interference from, in this case, radioactivity in tissues other than those in the image plane, image contrast is much higher than in planar imaging. It is primarily dependent upon the relative concentration of radioactivity in the structure of interest and adjacent tissue.

A.2.2.2 Applicability of the Proposed Technique for Measuring Image Quality. Many of the comments made about the potential applicability of the image quality assessment in relation to x-ray CT apply also to the single photon emission computed tomography. In measuring the quality of the acquired data, the effect of distance dependence of the camera's MTF must be taken into account, as must the fact that both noise and spatial resolution in the reconstructed image have a radial dependence.

The ROC methodology has been successfully used to assess the quality of the SPECT images for many years (*e.g.*, Carril *et al.*, 1979).

A.2.3 Positron Emission Tomography

A.2.3.1 Basic Imaging Technique. By labelling a pharmaceutical with a positron-emitting radionuclide, rather than a single gamma-ray emitter, it is possible to reconstruct the image by simultaneously detecting the pair of gamma-rays emitted back-to-back when the positron annihilates. By using a ring-shaped detector surrounding the patient, tomographic images can be produced by recording the almost simultaneous arrival of each pair of gammas. The point of origin of the radiation must then lie somewhere along the line joining these two recorded points. The three-dimensional information is derived from the points of intersection of many such rays. In a recent development, the very small difference in the

with the technique. A general overview of the topic is given by Brown *et al.* (1988).

The most promising results, perhaps, are those in which dynamic physiological activity (such as gastric emptying and lung ventilation) is being studied. It has yet to find a routine clinical application.

A.5.2.2 Applicability of the Proposed Technique for Measuring Image Quality. Electrical impedance images are nonlinear, shift variant and noise limited. This Report is concerned mainly with the impact of noise in signal detectability and to this extent the methods are applicable to electrical impedance imaging. At this stage in the development of the imaging technique, however, the intractability of the solution of the inverse problem is the primary limitation in imaging performance.

A.5.3 Biomagnetic Imaging

A.5.3.1 Basic Imaging Technique. Biological activity, particularly in the heart and the brain, is accompanied by the production of weak magnetic fields. Of course, it is well known that such biological activity can be studied by means of the electrocardiogram and the electroencephalogram recordings. The strongest of these magnetic signals is that due to cardiac activity [of the order of 50 pico Tesla (pT)]; the oculogram is around 10 pT, the encephalogram, 1 pT, and the visually evoked response as little as 0.2 pT.

The very weak magnetic fields that originate within the body can be detected by semiconductor quantum interference device (SQUID) gradiometers positioned outside the body. The sensitivity of the SQUID is limited by noise and it is essential to carry out the measurements in a shielded room. The production of the image involves the solution of the inverse problem. Although the magnetic field is not significantly affected by soft tissues, the full solution of the inverse problem requires the calculation of the magnitude, position and direction of all the individual magnetic vectors within the three-dimensional volume. Typically, an array of 37 SQUIDS is used to provide the data and signal averaging is employed for noise reduction unless it is important to observe isolated events.

The equipment required for this technique is very expensive and currently has no routine clinical application.

A.5.3.2 Applicability of the Proposed Technique for Measuring Image Quality. The spatial localization of magnetic sources within the body is analogous to radionuclide imaging with a gamma camera. The principal limit on imaging is set by the signal-to-noise ratio. In addition, there is marked shift variance over large image areas. The methods developed in this Report, however, are generally applicable to biomagnetic images.

A.5.4 Light Transmission Imaging

A.5.4.1 Basic Imaging Technique. The absorption and scattering of light is different in the various tissues of the body. Within the visible range, there is intense scattering and transmission imaging is impossible except with very thin tissue specimens. In the near infrared, however, attenuation is up to two orders of magnitude less and scattering is strongly forward peaked. Moreover, some biological materials (particularly haemoglobin) are relatively strong absorbers of infrared radiation so transmission images with high contrast can be obtained.

Imaging of accessible structures can be achieved by observing the shadow resulting from infrared illumination of the opposite side. The resolution depends upon the geometry of the structures being imaged. The principal problem is due to the scattered light which reduces target detectability. Because scattered photons arrive later than those which have travelled on the direct path, the contrast reduction due to scattering can be reduced by taking time-of-flight into account. This can be done either by transmitting a short pulse of light, or by modulating the amplitude of the light at a high frequency and comparing the phase of the received signal with a suitable reference.

The technique has been evaluated for screening for breast cancer but, to date, has been found to have an unacceptably high number of false positives.

A.5.4.2 Applicability of the Proposed Technique for Measuring Image Quality. The application of the techniques proposed in this Report to light transmission imaging suffers from the fact that it is neither linear nor shift invariant.

Appendix B
Image Degradation

The detailed mechanisms by which images are degraded are, of course, dependent on the imaging modality. There are, however, a number of important classes of degradation and these will now be discussed. It is important to note that some forms of degradation are reversible while others are not.

B.1 Spatial Resolution

In general, the signal detected at each point in an image is significantly correlated to those at nearby points and this effect limits the degree to which the detailed structure of the subject is recorded since these correlations tend to "blur" the image. The interaction between signals detected at nearby points, commonly referred to as the spatial resolution of an imaging system, can arise in a number of ways. For example, in conventional projection radiography, finite focal spot size and energy dispersion in the detector both contribute to loss of detail. In scintigraphy, the overlapping penumbra of adjacent collimator holes and uncertainty in the computation of position lead to a similar effect. In principle, lost detail can be substantially recovered if the nature of the degradation process is known, but the practicality of this approach is limited in the presence of noise.

B.2 Noise

Real imaging systems introduce a random, or noise, component into the acquired data. The uncertainty this represents can arise from fundamental physical limitations such as statistical fluctuations of the x-ray photon flux in conventional radiology or thermal background in magnetic resonance imaging. Noise can arise from instrumental factors such as the incomplete detection of the available signal or electronic/thermal noise in the detector system. Because of its random nature, the presence of noise fundamentally limits the degree to which knowledge of the subject can be recovered from the acquired data. The extent to which information will be lost by an imaging system can be analyzed by modelling the behavior of both the true signal and the noise. Such models can, in principle, also be used to partially correct for noise degradation by computing the most probable distribution from the observed data.

B.3 Geometric Distortion

Many image systems fail to preserve a simple geometrical relationship between the acquired data and the subject under investigation. For example, an image intensifier x-ray system may introduce pincushion distortion while refraction at surfaces can alter the geometry of ultrasound images. Predictable geometric distortion is not particularly serious since it can be easily corrected if exact knowledge of geometry is important to the application. Distortion which can vary with time, or which is dependent on the subject, is difficult to correct and may render quantitative analysis impractical.

B.4 Point Intensity Distortion

An imaging system requires a means of detecting the spatial distribution of signals from the subject. Preferably a detector would give a response proportional to the signal it receives, but many detectors achieve this, at best, for only a limited range of signal magnitude. For example, direct x-ray film may record a density proportional to x-ray exposure, but only up to some critical point beyond which the recorded density becomes steadily less sensitive to additional exposure. In addition, the response characteristics may vary from one part of the detector system to another. For example, a scintillation camera image of a uniform radioactive source will generally demonstrate non-uniformity. For applications where a knowledge of signal intensity is important, it is often possible to use a calibration object to establish the response characteristic at each point in the detector so that the ideal-detector data can be calculated from the observed data.

B.5 Quantization

Imaging systems, in general, do not work with continuous data. Sensed data and displayed images are normally represented by associating one of a finite number of intensity levels with each set of spatial samples. This is even true for x-ray film which is composed of silver halide grains, each of which, after exposure to radiation and development, can be either opaque or transparent. In digital systems (x-ray CT, MRI, digital subtraction angiograhy, etc.) intensity values are stored with limited numerical resolution for a regular array of sample points (pixels). The process of spatial and intensity quantization can lead to irretrievable loss of information. There are well-defined rules that specify the conditions which must be met in order to avoid such information loss, and it is essential that they be observed (see, *e.g.*, Pratt, 1991).

B.6 Mismatch to the Observer

The output of a medical imaging system is generally a display which is viewed by clinicians. Both live (video) and hard copy displays are used. It is quite common for information which has been successfully acquired to be lost to the observer at this stage due to a failure to match the characteristics of the display to the sensory system of the user. Amongst the more obvious mechanisms for information loss are false contouring, due to a failure to correctly interpolate sampled data, and mismatch in the spatial or intensity dynamic range.

B.7 Conclusion

Geometrical distortion, point intensity distortion and quantization loss can often either be relatively easily corrected or substantially avoided by careful system design. In contrast, the effects of spatial correlation, noise and mismatch to the observer are more fundamental. Thus, most studies of image quality deal with their effect.

Appendix C

The Ideal Bayesian Observer

C.1 Overview

This Appendix gives the mathematical derivation of the SNR_I (presented in Equation 3.10). The first section introduces the concept of using the likelihood ratio as a decision function to determine in which of two possible alternative categories an image belongs (*e.g.*, the patient's clinical condition being either normal or abnormal). It is then shown that, for the simple case of a task with SKE/BKE, where the only fluctuations in the data are due to noise, the likelihood ratio can be calculated from the image data, the system transfer function, the difference between the objects in the two possible categories and the inverse of the image noise power.

The likelihood ratio decision function may be implemented for this problem by weighting the image data with a simple template. The shape of the template is equal to the difference between the signal expected in the two cases, while the noise factor removes any correlations, or structure, that may be present in the noise, converting it (for the purpose of the analysis) to white noise. The decision as to which class the image belongs is then made on whether or not the output from the template exceeds a threshold value.

Finally, using the fact that the SNR is simply a measure of the overlap between the probability distributions corresponding to the possible values of the likelihood ratio in each of the two states, the SNR_I is derived. The equation for SNR_I is given both for the general case (Equation C.6) and when the imaging system is linear, shift invariant and the noise can be assumed to be additive (Equation C.8).

The reason for adopting this approach is that decisions based on the likelihood ratio give the highest possible ROC curve, *i.e.*, the ideal observer is one whose performance at analyzing the data cannot be bettered.

C.2 Mathematical Derivation of the Ideal Observer Signal-to-Noise Ratio

The ideal observer is the Bayesian decision maker who minimizes the cost or risk when determining a decision strategy for a given task. The ideal observer decision function is monotonically related to and, hence, completely equivalent to, the likelihood-ratio decision function. The most commonly considered task is that of simple hypothesis testing with two possible alternative categories, *e.g.*, "normal" (hypothesis H_1) vs. "abnormal" (hypothesis H_2) and, in fact,

corresponds to the kinds of tasks usually considered when test objects and phantoms are designed.

The decision maker is given the image data set, $\mathbf{g}$, and must decide which of two hypotheses, H_1 or H_2, is more compatible with this data set. The decision maker calculates the posterior "betting odds" for hypothesis H_2 vs. H_1: $p(H_2|\mathbf{g})/p(H_1|\mathbf{g})$. Bayes' theorem is then applied to give the posterior probabilities $p(H_k|\mathbf{g})$ in terms of the more readily calculable conditional probability distributions for the data given each hypothesis, $p(\mathbf{g}|H_k)$ (Fukunaga, 1972):

$$p(H_k|\mathbf{g}) = p(\mathbf{g}|H_k)p(H_k)/p(\mathbf{g}). \quad (C.1)$$

The ratio of these expressions under the two hypotheses is proportional to the likelihood ratio, L, which is, therefore, an equivalent decision function:

$$L = p(\mathbf{g}|H_2)/p(\mathbf{g}|H_1). \quad (C.2)$$

The likelihood ratio is a scalar random variable that depends on the random data values but not on the prior probabilities. Given a data set, the ideal observer chooses between the two hypotheses by forming the likelihood ratio and comparing it to a criterion, or threshold, saying H_2 is true if the likelihood ratio is above the threshold and H_1 is true if the likelihood ratio is below the threshold. Any monotonic function of L is exactly equivalent to the ideal decision function (L_I) and will result in the same functional relationship between true-positive and false-positive error rates. The hypothesis H_1 or H_2 is chosen depending on whether

$$L_I < L_c$$

or

$$L_I > L_c, \quad (C.3)$$

respectively, where L_c is the threshold or cut-off level set by the observer according to some criterion. One approach is to set L_c in order to minimize the expected decision cost, or, equivalently, to maximize expected utility (Green and Swets, 1966). Another approach is to set the cut-off level to meet a specified false-positive response rate and to compare systems based on the true-positive rates. More generally, the dependence of the TPF as a function of the FPF can be studied as this threshold is varied. The resulting function is called an ROC curve, and systems can then be compared based on their ROC curves (see Section 4).

The simplest type of decision task is the case where the signal and background in the object are known exactly (SKE/BKE) and the only fluctuations in the data **g** are due to noise. For a linear system transfer function **H** acting on an input signal **f** with additive, zero-mean, and Gaussian distributed noise, the data can be completely characterized by their mean values, $\bar{\mathbf{g}}_k = \mathbf{H}\mathbf{f}_k$, and their covariance matrix, $\mathbf{C}_{\mathbf{n}_k}$, under hypothesis H_k (see Section 3.2.3). For the commonly encountered case of $\mathbf{C}_{\mathbf{n}_1} = \mathbf{C}_{\mathbf{n}_2} = \mathbf{C}_{\mathbf{n}}$, *i.e.*, the noise is additive (independent of amplitude and therefore independent of hypothesis), the decision function is linear in **g** (Fukunaga, 1972):

$$L_I = (\mathbf{H}\Delta\mathbf{f})^t \mathbf{C}_{\mathbf{n}}^{-1} \mathbf{g}, \qquad (C.4)$$

where $\Delta\mathbf{f} = \mathbf{f}_2 - \mathbf{f}_1$, *i.e.*, the difference between the input signals under the two hypotheses, and the superscript t indicates the transpose. The ideal observer weights the data by the expected difference signal, *i.e.*, "looks most closely" where the expected difference in the data is greatest, and weights inversely by the noise. This is seen explicitly when the noise is uncorrelated, or "white," since then the correlation matrix and its inverse are diagonal, with $(\mathbf{C}_{\mathbf{n}}^{-1})_{jj} = (1/\sigma_{\mathbf{n}}^2)$. If, in addition, the noise is constant as a function of position, $\mathbf{C}_{\mathbf{n}}$ is proportional to the identity matrix, $\mathbf{C}_{\mathbf{n}} = \sigma_{\mathbf{n}}^2 \mathbf{I}$. The decision function becomes a simple template match as shown in Figure C.1. That is, the ideal observer constructs a template from the expected difference signal, places it over the region of the expected signal and multiplies the acquired data point-by-point with this template, accumulating the total sum as it goes along.

The decision, H_2 or H_1, is then made depending on whether this accumulated value is greater than or less than the criterion, or threshold setting, of the decision function. When the noise is correlated, the ideal decision maker uses knowledge of the noise correlations to decorrelate or "whiten" the noise. The above discussion then holds with respect to the whitened image.

It is now possible to calculate a figure of merit for the ideal decision maker. The decision variable has a distribution under each of the hypotheses; how much these distributions overlap determines how well the ideal observer will be able to correctly discriminate between data from the two hypotheses. A simple example is given in Figure C.2.

Ideal observer performance can be quantified by calculating the mean, $\langle L_I \rangle_k$, and variance, σ_k^2, of the decision variable L_I under each hypothesis, k = 1, 2. The Ideal Observer SNR squared, SNR_I^2, is then defined as the ratio of the square of the difference of the means to the average of the variances:

$$SNR_I^2 = \frac{[\langle L_I \rangle_2 - \langle L_I \rangle_1]^2}{\frac{1}{2}[\sigma_1^2 + \sigma_2^2]}. \qquad (C.5)$$

For example, for the case of Gaussian distributed noise and equal covariance matrices ($\mathbf{C}_{\mathbf{n}} = \mathbf{C}_{\mathbf{n}_1} = \mathbf{C}_{\mathbf{n}_2}$), the decision function L_I is linear in the data, so that it is also Gaussian distributed. The difference of the means turns out to be identical to the averaged variance; their cancellation leaves the SNR_I^2 equal to one power of the difference of the means, namely

$$SNR_I^2 = (\mathbf{H}\Delta\mathbf{f})^t \mathbf{C}_{\mathbf{n}}^{-1} (\mathbf{H}\Delta\mathbf{f}). \qquad (C.6)$$

Note how this may be either written in the image domain as $\Delta\bar{\mathbf{g}}^t \mathbf{C}_{\mathbf{n}}^{-1} \Delta\bar{\mathbf{g}}$ or in the object domain as $\Delta\mathbf{f}^t \mathbf{C}_{\mathbf{f}}^{-1} \Delta\mathbf{f}$ where $\mathbf{C}_{\mathbf{f}}^{-1} \equiv \mathbf{H}^t \mathbf{C}_{\mathbf{n}}^{-1} \mathbf{H}$ is the image noise covariance as referred to the object domain.

For stationary noise, it is usually more convenient to work in the spatial-frequency domain with the (inherently diagonal) noise power spectrum rather than in the spatial domain with the autocorrelation function. Therefore, most of the examples which are presented in this Report will be worked out in the spatial-frequency domain, where

$$\Delta\mathbf{f}^t \overset{FT}{\longleftrightarrow} \Delta\tilde{\mathbf{f}}^*, \mathbf{C}_{\mathbf{n}} \overset{FT}{\longleftrightarrow} \mathbf{W}_{\mathbf{n}}, \mathbf{g}^t \overset{FT}{\longleftrightarrow} \tilde{\mathbf{g}}^* \text{ and } \mathbf{H}^t \overset{FT}{\longleftrightarrow} K \cdot OTF^*,$$

with $\mathbf{W}_{\mathbf{n}}$ the noise power and OTF the optical transfer function (whose magnitude is the MTF).

The following are the notational conventions to be used here. When going from the present discrete representation (with matrix sums) to a continuous representation (with integrals) for the linear shift-invariant case with stationary noise, only a simple

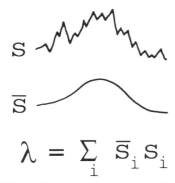

Fig. C.1. Schematic representation of a Gaussian matched filter testing for a signal, $\bar{s}$, in a noisy trace, s. The decision is based on whether the decision function, λ, exceeds the value of the decision threshold.

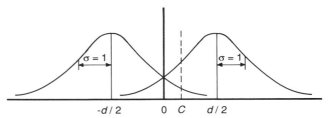

Fig. C.2. Distribution of the likelihood ratio decision variable for hypothesis H_2 (right) and H_1 (left). C is the decision criterion and d the separation of means of the two distributions in units of their common standard deviation.

notational modification will be made: The bold (matrix) notation will be unbolded, and an argument (in parentheses) will be added to the quantity; the quantity is then to be understood as a density. For example, for the case of stationary noise, the continuous noise power $\mathbf{W}$ will be modified to the noise power spectral density $W(\ )$. In addition, the continuous representation used throughout the Appendices will be extended to two or more dimensions by the use of bold arguments, $\mathbf{r}$ for spatial coordinates, and $\boldsymbol{\nu}$ for spatial frequency variables. The dimensionality of these vectors, and integrations carried out over them, will be obvious from the context.

Given that the stationary noise is diagonal in the spatial-frequency domain, $i.e.$, the frequency channels are independent, one may simply integrate over frequencies $\boldsymbol{\nu}$:

$$L_I = K \int \frac{\Delta \tilde{f}^*(\boldsymbol{\nu}) \mathrm{OTF}^*(\boldsymbol{\nu})}{W_n(\boldsymbol{\nu})} \tilde{g}(\boldsymbol{\nu}) \, d\boldsymbol{\nu}, \qquad (C.7)$$

where $\Delta \tilde{f}^*(\boldsymbol{\nu})$ is the complex conjugate Fourier transform of the difference between the signals under the two hypotheses. L_I is the so-called PWMF for the SKE/BKE task in additive Gaussian noise. The pre-whitening has the effect of playing down frequencies where the noise is greater, the $\Delta \tilde{f}^*(\boldsymbol{\nu})$ matching has the effect of playing up frequencies where the expected signal strength is greater; and the presence of the OTF factor in the weighting has the effect of modifying the expected signal strength according to how strongly it passes through the system. The ideal filter looks most keenly where the signal is most expected and least keenly where the noise is most expected. This basic principle carries through all of signal detection theory and statistical decision theory, although it may become more complicated as uncertainties in signal parameters are introduced.

It is now possible to calculate a figure of merit for the ideal decision maker in the frequency domain. This is obtained by calculating the mean and variance of the decision function L_I under both hypotheses, as was done in the spatial domain. Now, however, given independent frequency channels it is straightforward to carry out the calculation. Identifying $\tilde{g}(\boldsymbol{\nu})$ as the random variable and $K \Delta \tilde{f}^* \mathrm{OTF}^*(\boldsymbol{\nu}) / W_n(\boldsymbol{\nu})$ as its weighting factor in each frequency channel in the expression for L_I, the difference of means and average variance of the decision function in the frequency domain are once again identical and, from the form of Equation C.5, equal to SNR_I^2. Therefore, the figure of merit for the ideal decision maker in the frequency domain is:

$$\mathrm{SNR}_I^2 = K^2 \int \frac{|\Delta \tilde{f}(\boldsymbol{\nu})|^2 \mathrm{MTF}^2(\boldsymbol{\nu})}{W_n(\boldsymbol{\nu})} \, d\boldsymbol{\nu} \equiv d_{\mathrm{SKE}}'^2, \qquad (C.8a)$$

where MTF is the modulation transfer function. This result for a linear system may be adapted to nonlinear systems by replacing K with κ, or by working with relative quantities, or contrasts, and by adopting the small-signal approximations of Section 3.2.1. In the latter case one obtains

$$\mathrm{SNR}_I^2 = \gamma^2 \int \frac{|\Delta \tilde{f}_{\mathrm{rel}}(\boldsymbol{\nu})|^2 \mathrm{MTF}^2(\boldsymbol{\nu})}{(W_n(\boldsymbol{\nu}))_{\mathrm{rel}}} \, d\boldsymbol{\nu}, \qquad (C.8b)$$

where the subscript "rel" means the measured variable is normalized by its mean value over the small-signal operating range. The range of validity of this approximate result must be established for each application. The notation d'_{SKE} refers to the "detectability index" which, for this case, is the SNR_I for the SKE/BKE case. Other subscripts and superscripts are used with the symbol d depending upon the type of observer and method of obtaining the index (see Section 4.2.3).

Appendix D

Examples of the Application of the Ideal Observer to Medical Imaging

D.1 Introduction

In this Appendix, several examples of the application of the ideal observer which lead to familiar results will be presented. Consider the case shown in Figure D.1, where the null hypothesis is that background alone is present, at a level $f_1(\mathbf{r}) = \overline{Q}$; the signal-present hypothesis is that a pill-box lesion is present as shown. The pill-box has an incremental height $\Delta f(\mathbf{r}) = f_2(\mathbf{r}) - f_1(\mathbf{r}) = \Delta Q$ above the background within a circular cross section of area $a = \pi r_0^2$ where r_0 is the radius of the lesion. Consider first the case where the MTF is perfect, *i.e.*, MTF $(\nu_x, \nu_y) = 1$ for all spatial frequencies, ν_x, ν_y. For the case where the image has resulted from x or gamma rays, the power spectrum $W_n(\nu_x, \nu_y)$ of the Poisson noise background level is equal to $\overline{Q}$ and has the units of counts per unit area.

The pill-box profile $b_0(\mathbf{r})$ is simply the circle function with argument r/r_0, where r is the magnitude of $\mathbf{r}$, and is defined to be unity within a circle of radius r_0 and zero outside. The difference object is, therefore, given by

$$\Delta f(\mathbf{r}) = \Delta Q b_0(\mathbf{r}). \tag{D.1}$$

In the Fourier domain the pill-box lesion becomes

$$\tilde{\Delta f}(\boldsymbol{\nu}) = (\Delta Q a) S_a(\boldsymbol{\nu}) \tag{D.2}$$

where $S_a(\boldsymbol{\nu})$ has the shape of the Airy disc (Goodman, 1968), $a = \pi r_0^2$, and $S_a(\boldsymbol{\nu})$ has the convenient normalization that $S_a(\mathbf{0}) = 1$ and

$$\int S_a^2(\boldsymbol{\nu}) \, d\boldsymbol{\nu} = \frac{1}{a}. \tag{D.3}$$

Then the equation for SNR_I gives immediately

$$SNR_I^2 = \int \frac{|\tilde{\Delta f}(\boldsymbol{\nu})|^2 MTF^2(\boldsymbol{\nu})}{W_n(\boldsymbol{\nu})} \, d\boldsymbol{\nu} = \frac{(\Delta Q)^2 a}{\overline{Q}}$$
$$= C^2 \overline{Q} a, \tag{D.4}$$

where the contrast $C = \Delta Q / \overline{Q}$ and is some natural ratio in the object or emitted or transmitted radiation for most physical applications. Note that this is the SNR used by Rose (1973) and Schade (1964; 1975).

The NPS is a constant independent of frequency since, for Poisson noise, the autocorrelation function is a delta function, *i.e.*, no correlations. The level of this constant spectrum is then $W_n(\mathbf{0})$ and may be determined as follows. Consider the variance σ_{QA}^2 of estimates of the random variable QA obtained by taking contiguous samples of the count density through an integrating window of area A. This sampling of a Poisson process is itself a Poisson process and so the variance is equal to the mean $\overline{Q}A$. Then, since var $(aX) = a^2$ var (X), we may write

$$\sigma_Q^2 = \frac{\sigma_{QA}^2}{A^2} = \frac{\overline{Q}A}{A^2} = \frac{\overline{Q}}{A}. \tag{D.5}$$

The level of the corresponding white-noise power spectrum $W_n(\mathbf{0})$ is then such that its integral is equal to σ_Q^2:

$$\sigma_Q^2 = \int W_n S_A^2(\boldsymbol{\nu}) \, d\boldsymbol{\nu} = W_n \int S_A^2 \, d\boldsymbol{\nu} = \frac{\overline{Q}}{A} \tag{D.6}$$

where $S_A(\nu)$ is the shape function corresponding to the window A. The normalization of S_A is again such that $S_A(\mathbf{0}) = 1$: This means that sampling by the window preserves counts. Therefore,

$$\int S_A^2(\boldsymbol{\nu}) \, d\boldsymbol{\nu} = \frac{1}{A} \tag{D.7}$$

and the level of the NPS is thus seen to be $W_n(\mathbf{0}) = \overline{Q}$.

If the difference object Δf in the example above is a two-dimensional Gaussian $[G_0(\mathbf{r})]$ profile with the RMS σ_0 and maximum height ΔQ, and the background f_1 taken to be a uniform level of $\overline{Q}$ counts per unit area (Figure D.2), *i.e.*, $f_2(\mathbf{r}) = \Delta Q G_0(\mathbf{r}) + \overline{Q}$ and $f_1(r) = \overline{Q} = W_n$, then the equivalent form for SNR_I becomes

$$SNR_I^2 = (C/2)^2 \overline{Q} a_0, \tag{D.8}$$

where $a_0 = 4\pi \sigma_0^2$ and $C = \Delta Q / \overline{Q}$. The Gaussian weighting has reduced SNR^2 by a factor of four (for this convention, see Wagner and Brown, 1985).

Now consider the more general case where the pre-noise-insertion MTF of the imaging system is not equal to unity, *i.e.*, it is not perfect. In this case, it is said that the imaging system "aperture" degrades the signal detectability. As an example of the aperture's role, consider the Gaussian signal degraded by an aperture, *e.g.*, x-ray tube focal spot, with transfer function

$$MTF(\boldsymbol{\nu}) = \exp(-2\pi^2 \sigma_{AP}^2 \nu^2), \tag{D.9}$$

where ν is the magnitude of $\boldsymbol{\nu}$. (The details of the geometrical scaling of this aperture and that of the image receptor to the object plane of interest are ignored here; this is treated by Wagner, 1977b).

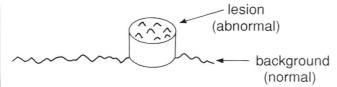

Fig. D.1. The task is to distinguish whether a pill-box lesion is present in a noisy background.

Straightforward substitution of Equation D.9 into Equation C.8 yields

$$\mathrm{SNR}_I^2 = \left\{\frac{C}{2}\right\}^2 \frac{\overline{Q}a_0^2}{a_0 + a_{AP}} = \left\{\frac{C}{2}\right\}^2 \frac{\overline{Q}a_0}{[1 + (a_{AP}/a_0)]}, \quad (D.10)$$

where the power spectral density is again equal to $\overline{Q}$, independent of frequency, since the system aperture is defined as a blur function which does not correlate, or color, the noise. As with the Gaussian object function $a_{AP} = 4\pi\sigma_{AP}^2$. An interesting and fundamental interpretation of this result comes from comparing it with the SNR for the case $f_2(\mathbf{r}) = P + S + \Delta P G_0(\mathbf{r})$, $f_1(\mathbf{r}) = P + S$, where P represents the primary fluence and S the scatter fluence. By direct substitution of ΔP for ΔQ and $P + S$ for $\overline{Q}$ into Equation D.8, it is straightforward to obtain for that case (Wagner *et al.*, 1980):

$$\mathrm{SNR}_{SC}^2 = \frac{(\Delta P)^2 a_0}{4(P + S)} = \left\{\frac{C}{2}\right\}^2 \frac{P a_0}{[1 + (S/P)]}, \quad (D.11)$$

where the contrast C is $\Delta P/P = \Delta\mu x$, *i.e.*, the line integral of the attenuation coefficient difference between signal and background, for the low contrast case. Now it can be seen that the role of the aperture in the above SNR_I is the same as the role played by the scatter term in SNR_{SC}, *i.e.*, the aperture degrades SNR by coupling signal to additional background noise in the way that the presence of scatter degrades SNR by coupling signal to additional background noise counts.

This has been the most elementary example of how the quantity $\mathrm{MTF}^2(\boldsymbol{\nu})/W(\boldsymbol{\nu})$ plays a central part in almost all SNRs encountered. This is because it is essentially the inverse of the noise in the data $\mathbf{g}(\mathbf{r})$, referred back to the input domain (see, *e.g.*, Equation

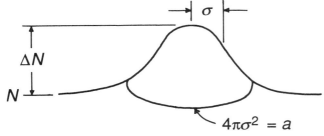

Fig. D.2. Low contrast Gaussian signal of height ΔQ above the background level $\overline{Q}$ and rms radius σ.

C.6 and comments following). Four different applications to practical imaging systems will now be considered to show how the combination of imaging measurements contained in this quantity serves as a unique specification of the system hardware at some particular operating level (exposure, time, etc.) of interest.

D.2 Example I. Screen/Film Systems and Photon Detection with Logarithmic Amplification

In the case of a screen/film system, there is a macroscopic transfer function that relates changes in the logarithm of the exposure, Q, to changes in output density, D. The slope of this transfer function is called the photographic gamma (γ) and is defined by the equation

$$\Delta D = \gamma\Delta(\log Q) = 0.434\gamma\Delta Q/\overline{Q}, \quad (D.12)$$

where 0.434 is $\log_{10} e$, and the second equality holds strictly only for low contrast. Notice that this definition of γ is consistent with that given earlier under the discussion of large-area transfer characteristics. This follows since the photographic density, $D = -\log T$, where T is the film transmission. The factor γ therefore represents the contrast gain from input Q to output T.

More generally, one must consider the combination of the macroscopic amplification with the microscopic degradation in resolution described by the modulation transfer function $\mathrm{MTF}(\boldsymbol{\nu})$. This yields the generalization of the macroscopic γ to the microscopic CTF (contrast transfer function) as

$$\Delta D(\boldsymbol{\nu}) = 0.434\mathrm{CTF}\Delta Q/\overline{Q}$$
$$= 0.434\gamma\mathrm{MTF}(\nu)\Delta Q/\overline{Q}. \quad (D.13)$$

This might also be written

$$\mathrm{d}(\Delta D)/\mathrm{d}(\Delta Q/\overline{Q}) = 0.434\gamma\mathrm{MTF}(\boldsymbol{\nu}). \quad (D.14)$$

In the simple example of Appendix D.1, the NPS for fluctuations of the exposure density Q on an absolute scale was shown, by invoking an integrating window, to be equal to $\overline{Q}$. If we again study the fluctuations of contiguous samples taken by an integrating window of area A, but now measured on a relative scale, we need only notice that

$$\sigma_{\Delta Q/\overline{Q}}^2 \equiv \sigma_{Q/\overline{Q}}^2 = \frac{\sigma_Q^2}{\overline{Q}^2} = \frac{1}{\overline{Q}^2}\frac{\overline{Q}}{A} = \frac{1}{\overline{Q}A} \quad (D.15)$$

$$W_{\Delta Q/\overline{Q}} \equiv W_{Q/\overline{Q}} = \frac{W_Q}{\overline{Q}^2} = \frac{\overline{Q}}{\overline{Q}^2} = \frac{1}{\overline{Q}} \quad (D.16)$$

The notation ΔQ refers to the fluctuations of Q about its mean value. The first equalities are therefore definitions and the remaining equalities follow immediately from Equations D.5 and D.6.

The measured output fluctuations are generally expressed in terms of the power spectrum of the density fluctuations on a film:

$$W_n(\boldsymbol{\nu}) = W_{\Delta D}(\boldsymbol{\nu}). \qquad (D.17)$$

If there was a perfect logarithmic recorder of photon fluctuations, then the power spectrum of those fluctuations would be:

$$W_{\Delta D}(\boldsymbol{\nu}) = (0.434)^2 \gamma^2 / \overline{Q}. \qquad (D.18)$$

This is simply the result of transferring a variance through a constant multiplier. (It is noteworthy that even if this recorder did not have a perfect MTF, the result would be the same as long as the MTF was strictly a pre-noise-insertion transfer function, *e.g.*, from such effects as x-ray focal spot blurring.) One could then deduce the number of exposure quanta involved in the detection process by measuring $W_{\Delta D}(\nu)$ and γ, *i.e.*,

$$\overline{Q} = \frac{(0.434)^2 \gamma^2}{W_{\Delta D}(\boldsymbol{\nu})}. \qquad (D.19)$$

However, in practice, there are other sources of output noise associated with the degradation in photon statistics by the imaging system including its inability to collect all of the input quanta. For this practical case, we *define* the number of noise equivalent quanta, $NEQ(\boldsymbol{\nu})$, as

$$NEQ(\boldsymbol{\nu}) = \frac{(0.434)^2 \gamma^2 MTF^2(\boldsymbol{\nu})}{W_{\Delta D}(\boldsymbol{\nu})}. \qquad (D.20)$$

The factors in the numerator of this equation are required to correctly refer the measured noise from the density domain through the overall transfer characteristics of the imaging system, namely, $\gamma MTF(\boldsymbol{\nu})$. This is a case of simply following the procedure put forth above of referring the covariance in the data back to the input (cf. Equation C.6).

With a logarithmic detector, relative changes in the input are being measured. This means that the mean signal must also be calibrated in relative exposure units, $\Delta Q / \overline{Q}$, as the fluctuations were just treated. For photon imaging systems working in a transmission mode, *e.g.*, planar radiography, this is the customary mode of operation. In the low contrast limit in which the assumption of additive Gaussian noise holds, it is also found that the relative change in transmitted quanta $\Delta Q / \overline{Q}$, due to the inclusion of a lesion material of thickness t within a large phantom of otherwise uniform transmission, is equal to $\Delta \mu t$, where $\Delta \mu$ is the difference in linear attenuation coefficient between the uniform phantom and the included lesion (Wagner, 1977b).

$NEQ(\boldsymbol{\nu})$ is the number of quanta the image is "worth" based on the image performance measurements, γ, $MTF(\boldsymbol{\nu})$ and $W(\boldsymbol{\nu})$. The image was actually made with $\overline{Q}$ exposure quanta but it is as if only NEQ of them show up in the image (Dainty and Shaw, 1974). The ratio $NEQ(\boldsymbol{\nu})/\overline{Q}$ is referred to as the detective quantum efficiency, DQE, of the imaging system and is, in general, a function of the operating point (exposure level, time, etc.). In Figure D.3, the values of $NEQ(\boldsymbol{\nu})$ as a function of spatial frequency for three calcium tungstate systems exposed to a film density of unity are given. These results are also shown in Figure D.3, normalized to the actual expo-

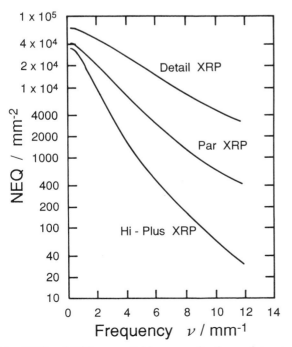

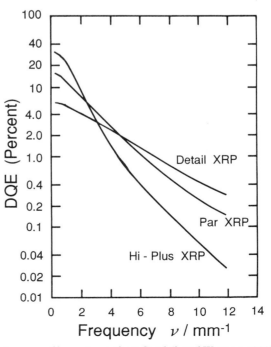

Fig D.3. NEQ and DQE vs. spatial frequency for three calcium tungstate screen-film systems (from Sandrik and Wagner, 1982).

sure quanta, $\overline{Q}$, required to achieve a unit density. This is the DQE(ν) spectrum. Notice that if the performance criterion is SNR or signal detection sensitivity (as measured by the NEQ), then the Detail system would be preferred. However, if the performance criterion is exposure efficiency—*i.e.*, efficient use of the exposure quanta Q— then the crossing of the DQE curves leads to an ambiguity: at low spatial frequencies, the Hi-Plus system would be preferred whereas at high spatial frequencies the Detail system would be preferred.

Typical screen/film systems exposed to unit film density have low-frequency NEQ values in the neighborhood of 4×10^4 counts · mm^{-2}. At lower and higher film densities, or lower and higher exposures, this value falls off due to the disproportionate contribution to the film noise from the film's own granularity near the low-exposure threshold and high-exposure saturation points. This is seen in the results shown in Figure D.4 for the Par-speed system. It is generally thought that screen/film systems have a dynamic range of about two orders of magnitude; if the NEQ or the DQE spectra are considered, however, then these systems are seen to have closer to only one order of magnitude of dynamic range.

A number of manufacturers have begun making such information available in the form of three-dimensional displays with accompanying contour maps. An example for the case of a mammographic screen-film system is given in Figure D.5.

When only the values of DQE are explicitly pre-sented, the corresponding values of NEQ can be obtained by exponentiating log Q, and then multiplying by DQE. For example, the maximum DQE in Figure D.5 corresponds to a value of Q of approximately $10^{5.5}$, or 3.2×10^5 photons · mm^{-2}; a low frequency value for DQE of 22 percent will then yield a value of NEQ of 0.7×10^5 photons · mm^{-2} for that region of the parameter space.

Note that in arriving at the expression for NEQ(ν), the MTF and the noise power spectrum enter independently; no assumption is made concerning a relation between the shape of the NPS and the squared MTF; that is, no model is being used here. It is simply a question of implementing the prescription for scaling the noise back to the object or input domain.

The formulation given above for photographic detection systems applies directly to other systems that use logarithmic detection. For purely logarithmic detection (base e), the equivalent gamma is unity and the constant $\log_{10}e$ does not enter in.

D.3 Example II. Linear Amplification: Image Intensifier Tubes/Nuclear Medicine Gamma Cameras

Consider next the effective noise at the input of a linear shift-invariant system

$$W_{in}^{-1}(\nu) = K^2 \text{MTF}^2(\nu)/W_n(\nu), \qquad (D.21)$$

where the W_{in}^{-1} notation was discussed in Section 3.4.

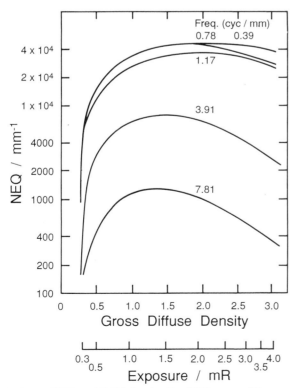

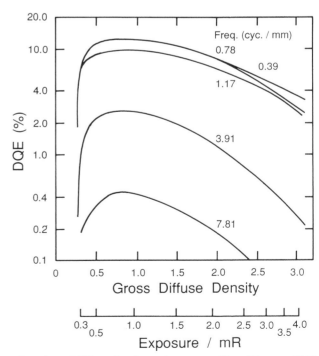

Fig. D.4. NEQ and DQE for the Par/XRP screen/film system as a function of diffuse density and exposure (from Wagner, 1983 and courtesy of J.M. Sandrick).

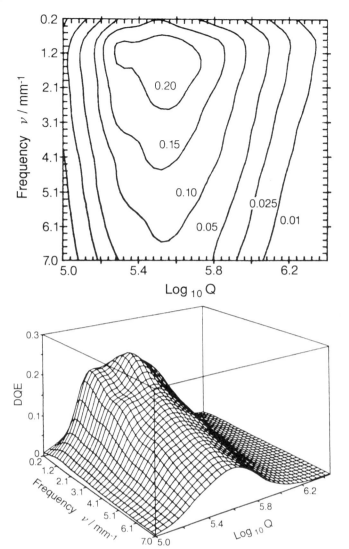

Fig. D.5. Detective quantum efficiency as a function of spatial frequency and log exposure (Log Q) for a mammographic screen-film system (absolute scale for Q is in photons $\cdot$ mm^{-2}) (from Bunch *et al.*, 1987).

This is relevant to the case of image intensifier tubes, nuclear medicine gamma cameras, and similar devices designed to give an output signal that is directly proportional to the input signal. In this case, $W_{\Delta Q}(\nu) = \overline{Q}$ at the input if $\overline{Q}$ is the average number of quanta per unit area incident on the detector. If the fluctuations were measured with a perfect detector with noise-free amplification, K, the measured power spectrum at the output would be $W_n(\nu) = K^2\overline{Q}$ (even for the non-unit pre-noise-insertion MTF, as above). However, any practical detector system will produce a spectrum of fluctuations that is worse than this value on an absolute scale. By analogy with the previous section, but now on an absolute scale as opposed to the logarithmic or relative scale, the equivalent number of detected quanta $\overline{Q}'$ is defined as

$$1/\overline{Q}'(\nu) = K^2MTF^2(\nu)/W_n(\nu). \qquad (D.22)$$

For the perfect system, one would obtain

$$1/\overline{Q}' = 1/\overline{Q}, \qquad (D.23)$$

but, in practice, one would find $\overline{Q}' > \overline{Q}$. In contrast to logarithmic amplification, where more photons produce less noise, now it is found that more photons give more noise, so the more noise, the more equivalent photons. That is, one is working on an absolute scale rather than the relative scale which arose from the log amplification.

To elaborate slightly, in any practical system there is more noise (especially in the case of an image intensifier or an intensifier/video system) than the Poisson noise of the photons and thus the value of W_n will increase. If one attempts to interpret the noise in terms of photons, one will get the impression that the number of photons has increased, which might mislead one to conclude that the system looks better. Therefore, some measure of normalization must be used. Once again that privileged normalization is in terms of the perfect detector for which $K^2MTF^2 = K^2$ and for which the noise power spectrum is equal to $K^2\overline{Q}$ at all frequencies. Then the DQE would be

$$DQE(\nu) = \overline{Q}/\overline{Q}'(\nu) \qquad (D.24)$$

compared to

$$DQE(\nu) = NEQ(\nu)/\overline{Q}, \qquad (D.25)$$

for the logarithmic detection, or screen-film, case.

One therefore would wish to measure the input exposure quanta, Q, the MTF and the NPS, $W_n(\nu)$, and present these results separately. For the purposes of determining the system efficiency, the DQE ratio is presented. For purposes of calculating the noise equivalent quantity that is used in the signal detection integrals, the DQE must be divided by the actual exposure quanta used, and the result of Equation D.22 will be recovered.

D.4 Example III. Magnetic Resonance Imaging/Fourier Domain Data Acquisition

In MRI, the data is acquired in the Fourier domain, and images are then produced by a 2D Fourier transform of this data. This transformation is simply the two-dimensional extension of the one-dimensional version used earlier. Because of the orthogonality properties of the Fourier transform, a very elementary form results for the NPS and, hence, for SNR_I^2 as shown below.

Thermal noise is the dominant source of noise in magnetic resonance imaging. It is generated in the effective resistance, R_e, of the patient and the receiving coil (Hoult and Lauterbur, 1979). The noise variance for each (voltage) measurement is $4kTR_e\Delta f_t$ where k is Boltzmann's constant, T is the absolute temperature and Δf_t is the bandwidth of the receiver.

In addition, the front-end amplification will degrade this by its noise figure, F_a, to $(4kTR_e\Delta f_t)F_a$.

For imaging in 2D, a 2D distribution of net magnetic moment $\rho(x, y)$ will be considered. The object of the MRI system is to determine the distribution of spins or spin density in the spatial domain from a set of measurements in the temporal-frequency/pseudo-temporal-frequency (phase encoded) domain, which is easily converted to the spatial-frequency domain $\tilde{\rho}(\nu_x, \nu_y)$, from a knowledge of the spatial-encoding gradients. Since the noise variance is given per measurement, it is convenient to use a discrete Fourier transform representation:

$$\rho(x, y) = \Sigma \, \tilde{\rho}(\nu_x, \nu_y) \exp\left[-2\pi i(\nu_x x + \nu_y y)\right]\Delta\nu_x\Delta\nu_y \quad \text{(D.26)}$$

$$\tilde{\rho}(\nu_x, \nu_y) = \Sigma \, \rho(x, y) \exp\left[2\pi i(\nu_x x + \nu_y y)\right]\Delta x\Delta y. \quad \text{(D.27)}$$

Since the thermal noise is white, or uncorrelated, one can write for the covariance of the measurements

$$\langle \delta\tilde{\rho}(\boldsymbol{\nu})\delta\tilde{\rho}(\boldsymbol{\nu}')\rangle = \delta_{\nu_x\nu_x'}\delta_{\nu_y\nu_y'}(4kTR_e\Delta f_t)F_a, \quad \text{(D.28)}$$

where the δ-functions on the right-hand side are to be interpreted as Kronecker delta functions.

The covariance in the image can be derived from this using the Fourier transform relations, Equations D.26 and D.27, and noticing that the spatial frequency cell has dimensions $\Delta\nu_x = 1/X$, $\Delta\nu_y = 1/Y$ when the region scanned has dimensions X and Y. If there is no smoothing of the image, the image noise will also be uncorrelated, and it is straightforward to show that the power spectrum in the image domain is (Wagner and Brown, 1985)

$$W(\boldsymbol{\nu}) = \frac{(4kTR_e\Delta f_t)F_a}{XY}, \quad \text{(D.29)}$$

independent of spatial frequency. If there is smoothing of the image, then the power spectrum is simply modified as described in Section 3.2.3.1 if the smoothing function is known.

The SNR for an imaging task with difference spectrum $\Delta\tilde{f}(\boldsymbol{\nu})$ can now be found:

$$\text{SNR}_I^2 = \int \frac{\Delta\tilde{f}^2(\boldsymbol{\nu})\tilde{H}^2(\boldsymbol{\nu})XY}{4kTR_e\Delta f_t F_a} \, d\boldsymbol{\nu}. \quad \text{(D.30)}$$

It can now be shown how this expression can be used to find the SNR_I^2 when the signal is an elevated pill-box of spins, as in the nuclear medicine example. Assume a flat background of spins which generates a two-dimensional signal of V volts per unit area. Against that background stands a pill-box signal which generates $V + \Delta V$ volts per unit area over an area $A = \pi r^2$. We may take the MTF to be equal to

unity for this example (and in fact in most MRI clinical practice the resolution limitations come from finite sampling effects). In the same way as for the SNR^2 for the pill-box lesion in the nuclear medicine example above, it is found that

$$\text{SNR}_I^2 = \int \frac{\Delta V^2 A^2 S_A^2(\boldsymbol{\nu})XY}{4kTR_e\Delta f_t F_a} \, d\boldsymbol{\nu}$$
$$= \frac{\Delta V^2 AXY}{4kTR_e\Delta f_t F_a} \quad \text{(D.31)}$$

since

$$\int S_A^2(\boldsymbol{\nu}) \, d\boldsymbol{\nu} = \frac{1}{A}. \quad \text{(D.32)}$$

In general one does not know the absolute efficiency of the coupling of spins to a voltage signal in the receiving coil. Therefore, in addition to the neglect of the effect of relaxation times on the signal strength in this analysis, there is also the neglect of an overall efficiency factor that, in principle, could be calibrated.

In practice, there will be more noise than the limiting value of the thermal noise used above. It will be necessary to measure the true noise power spectrum and use it in place of the quantity $4kTR_e\Delta f_t F_a$. (In practice, this may be more difficult than it might seem because of the lack of reproducibility in phase-encode errors and the presence of additional artifacts.) One may then proceed by analogy with the photon imaging procedures given above: the measurement bandwidth is generally known; from the noise power spectrum measurement, and knowledge of this bandwidth, one may deduce an equivalent temperature-resistance product, TR_e, if the noise figure F_a is known, or an equivalent product TR_eF_a if it is not known. These results may be used to calculate the detective quantum efficiency if values of the temperature and resistance under ideal conditions can be identified. Until this point is reached, it is of interest to compare the noise of various systems on a relative scale (percent).

The SNR^2 given here for MRI describes the performance for one complete set of phase encodes. Generally, images are acquired and averaged over several such sets. The number of sets is referred to as the number of excitations, N_{ex}, and should be included as a multiplicative factor in Equation D.31. In addition, discrete effects such as the number and spacing of phase encodes and spacing of samples within each phase encoded data trace will need to be included to adapt the continuous treatment given here to the discrete case.

The NMR signal, of course, does not just depend on the density of spins in the sample. MRI achieves its great soft tissue discriminating power due to the weighting of the spin densities by the natural relaxation times and the measurement times involved in data acquisition. Magnetic resonance imaging contrast has been reviewed in detail by Edelstein *et al.* (1983). In practice, the signal contrast must be measured using a phantom with known and stable parameters. Finally, the absolute signal strength in volts and its scaling to machine or image numbers must be determined by calibration measurements if the SNR is desired on an absolute scale.

When the SNR^2 is calculated at the pixel level, a peculiar property of MRI SNR^2 emerges: it depends on the square of the pixel area. In photon projection imaging, this dependence was found to be according to the first power of the pixel area, leading to the possibility of integrating pixels to exactly recover SNR from finely sampled pixels (ignoring system aperture limitations). In MRI, this quadratic dependence on pixel area leads to irretrievable SNR loss when the pixel size is reduced (Edelstein *et al.*, 1986).

In the same light, it should be pointed out that the expression for the SNR^2 shows a handicap of NMR-zoom where the entire bandwidth Δf_t is spread over only a limited region of the format XY, thereby reducing the numerator in Equation D.31.

D.5 Example IV. Images Reconstructed from Projections — Computed Tomography and Positron Emission Tomography

Central to an understanding of CT is a fundamental theorem of two-dimensional Fourier analysis called the central-slice theorem. An heuristic derivation of this theorem with its simple interpretation will be given. First, consider two-dimensional MRI where the data are acquired in two dimensions in a domain that is essentially the spatial frequency domain of the required image. The data acquisition is such that this two-dimensional frequency space is sampled on a uniformly spaced two-dimensional Cartesian grid or lattice. In CT, however, the two-dimensional frequency domain is essentially sampled on a two-dimensional polar grid (see Figure D.6a). To see this, assume that the first view in a CT system is made up of line integrals along transverse rays through the head of the patient (Figure D.6b). When the one-dimensional Fourier transformation of the line-integral data is taken, it yields a slice of the two-dimensional Fourier transformation of the image of the head. In the direction along the rays, the zero-frequency or DC component automatically results since the line integral is essentially the average or sum of the attenuation along the path. This one-dimensional Fourier transformation is therefore a slice, or spoke, of the two-dimensional transformation that runs through the center of spatial-frequency space. It characterizes the appropriate range of one-dimensional spatial frequencies along the spoke, and zero spatial-frequency orthogonal to the spoke. When the next view is taken, the argument just given is repeated, but with the coordinate system rotated by the angular shift between views. In this way, CT essentially builds up a 2D sampling of frequency space on a polar grid as in the figure. Even though the acquired data is usually not Fourier transformed, these statements are rigorous with respect to the effective sampling in the Fourier domain. One can see, then, that frequency space is sampled most densely at the origin and the sampling falls off like a radial pattern of spokes, that is, with a $1/\nu$ fall-off. Here, ν is the magnitude of the spatial frequency in the radial direction. The "filter" in filtered back-projection is therefore designed to effectively compensate for this deficiency in sampling at higher frequencies. In the frequency domain it is referred to as a ramp or ν filter.

The problem of signal detection theory in CT and

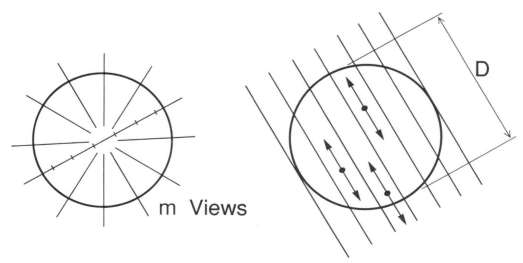

Fig. D.6. (a) Frequency domain geometry for ray projection tomography, with one slice corresponding to a given projection (with tick marks) and other rays indicating other projection angles. (b) Spatial domain geometry showing strip integrals (and positron annihilation events - *a propos* PET) for a single projection.

other imaging modalities using two-dimensional reconstruction from projections can be addressed at two levels. First, one may consider exclusively the actual detected projection data, since that is all the ideal observer would need to work with. On the other hand, the investigator studying the assessment of images will need to analyze the reconstructed image data since that is presented for analysis. The development for both approaches will be carried out and the connection between them noted.

First, consider x-ray CT where the attenuation coefficient of the phantom or body is the quantity of interest. Since the attenuation is exponential, the first stage of CT detection is logarithmic, with log to the base e. The power spectrum of detected signals is derived as in the screen/film case, but in this case all of the normalization factors reduce to unity. That is, the power spectrum for one view in CT is $1/\overline{Q}$, where $\overline{Q}$ is the (linear) density of detected counts along the periphery of the phantom or body, in one view. For m views (over 180°), the power spectrum of detected counts is scaled by the factor $F_1 = m/\pi\nu$, i.e., there are $2m$ rays uniformly distributed over an annulus of length $2\pi\nu$ at any radius, ν, in frequency space (see Figure D.6b).

Now, however, if the power spectrum as measured in the reconstructed image is needed, the CT reconstruction algorithm must be considered. As discussed above, the standard image reconstruction algorithm in CT has the shape of a ramp in frequency space; and the detected noise power spectrum will be scaled proportionally to the absolute square of a ramp, namely ν^2. With the correct normalization required for quantitative reconstructions, this becomes the factor $(\pi\nu/m)^2 = 1/F_1^2$. These results are summarized in Table D.1. For the reconstructed image there is an additional factor, called MTF_{alg}^2, which is the square of the transfer function that characterizes the smooth roll-off of the reconstruction algorithm at high frequencies.

Just as the CT case is analogous to the screen/film case or logarithmic amplification example, the application to PET is analogous to the nuclear medicine or linear amplification example given above. The power spectrum is linearly proportional to the mean density of detected counts along the periphery of the object, $\overline{Q}$. However, we must relate this to the mean two-dimensional density of activity in the object or phantom, $\overline{\rho}$, and the overall diameter of the phantom, D. Assuming no attenuation in the phantom, perfect collimation and detection, we find $\overline{Q} = \overline{\rho}D$. This may be scaled for attenuation if desired. The effects of multiple views, and of the reconstruction algorithm, are handled exactly as in the CT case and the results are presented in Table D.1.

In a practical measurement on a real imaging system, not all of the radiation incident on the detectors will contribute to the image, and there may be additional noise from the detection stage. It is for this reason that the DQE was defined, in Section D.2, in terms of the ratio of the image's worth, NEQ, to the actual mean number of radiation quanta, $\overline{Q}$, incident upon the detectors. In CT, a simple graphical construction technique using the image measurements of MTF and W yields the DQE or actual NEQ that replaces the value of $\overline{Q}$ in the table for any practical CT system (Wagner *et al.*, 1979). In the process, the blurring effects of the system hardware, in particular the pre-noise-insertion focal spot and detector aperture, referred to as MTF_{na} or the non-algorithmic MTF, can be separated from the post-noise-insertion blurring due to the software, namely MTF_{alg}.

The construction is based on the fact that the

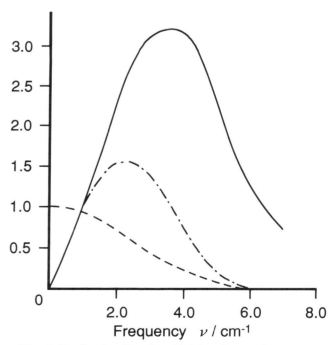

Fig. D.7. Construction for obtaining the aperture or non-algorithmic MTF^2 for a second generation CT scanner. The total system MTF^2, weighted for two dimensions by multiplying it by ν, is shown by curve -·-·-·. This is then divided by the normalized noise power spectrum, curve ——, to give the non-algorithmic MTF^2 curve - - - -. The ordinate has units of spatial frequency except for the aperture MTF^2, which is dimensionless (from Wagner *et al.*, 1979).

TABLE D.1—*Noise power spectra for images reconstructed from projections* ($F_1 = m/\pi\nu$)

	CT	PET
Data	$F_1/\overline{Q}$	$\overline{\rho}\Delta F_1$
Image	$(F_1/\overline{Q})MTF_{alg}^2(1/F_1)^2 =$	$(\overline{\rho}DF_1)MTF_{alg}^2(1/F_1)^2 =$
	$(\pi\nu/m\,\overline{Q})MTF_{alg}^2$	$\overline{\rho}D(\pi\nu/m)MTF_{alg}^2$

measured system MTF, namely MTF_{tot}, contains the product of MTF_{na} and MTF_{alg}; the measured noise, however, contains only the effect of the software blurring, MTF_{alg}. Also, to be commensurate with two-dimensional image noise, the one-dimensional $\text{MTF}^2_{\text{tot}}$ — a one-dimensional quantity — must be multiplied by a factor ν to have the correct two-dimensional frequency space weighting.

The construction is shown in Figure D.7. By dividing the noise power spectrum into the properly weighted total system MTF^2, the MTF^2 of the hardware results. The hardware MTF is simply the frequency space representation of the blur function in the original projections. Only this blurring is fundamental: it determines the region over which signal counts are dispersed among background counts, with the concomitant increase in noise and decrease in the SNR discussed above for conventional radiography. The size of this region ranged from 1 to 2 mm for the first and second generation head scanners. This is called the "terminal blur" since its effect on the SNR cannot be removed by image processing, although this has been attempted periodically.

When this construction and division are carried out on an absolute scale, they yield the NEQ spectrum for CT that is totally analogous to the NEQ spectrum for conventional radiography discussed above. This NEQ contains contributions from all m views and is comparable to $m\overline{Q}$ in the table. The absolute scale for the ordinate of the second generation system is given on Figure D.7 as $1 \equiv 1.8 \times 10^8$ cm^{-1} along the projections. [NEQ for CT is given as a linear density because CT averages over the cut (axial) direction; since the latter is usually about 1 cm, the aereal density is about the same.] In Figure D.8, the NEQ spectrum for the first generation CT system is given; the absolute scale for the ordinate here is 1.4×10^8 cm^{-1}. It can be seen, therefore, that the second generation represented both an increase in NEQ level and an increase in NEQ bandwidth — both achieved

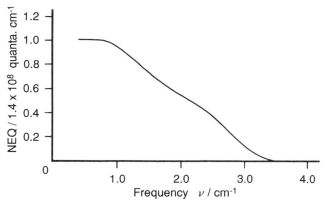

Fig. D.8. Noise equivalent quanta vs. frequency for a first generation CT system (from Wagner *et al.*, 1979).

without an increase in dose. Finally, it should be pointed out that these CT scans (head mode) were made with a total of almost 10^{10} effective detected counts. It is this great number that allows CT to make the subtle gray matter/white matter distinction in images of the brain.

The absolute scale in the analysis just given is achieved by noting that the total noise variance is in units of (CT number)^2, and equating the difference in CT number between air and water to approximately 0.19 cm^{-1}, the total attenuation coefficient of water at the beam quality used in these systems. The analysis then gives NEQ in units of cm^{-1}.

The DQE of CT can be determined in a manner similar to that for conventional images. In Wagner *et al.* (1979) it was found that the large-area or low-frequency NEQ represented approximately 65 percent of the exposure quanta for the EMI Mark I first generation CT, *i.e.*, the low frequency DQE = 0.65; or the large-area information in the image represented 65 percent of the information incident on the detectors. This was remarkable in the face of promises from some members of the mathematical community working on CT algorithms that they could reduce CT dose by an order of magnitude. In fact, at that time it was possible through improvements in hardware to reduce CT dose further since the beam collimation was poor. In the second generation system, only about one-third of the downstream beam was intercepted by the detectors. The dose efficiency of second generation CT was, therefore, estimated to be approximately $0.65 \times 0.33 = 0.22$. An independent estimate by Hanson (1979b; 1981) placed the efficiency between 0.12 and 0.17. Since that time, low dose collimation has been introduced, and, in principle, it has become possible to carry out CT at better than 50 percent total dose efficiency.

Examples will now be given comparing PET and time-of-flight PET (TOFPET) by calculating the lesion SNR in the acquired data or projections. Consider the problem of detecting a lesion with a 2D Gaussian profile (mean square length in any single dimension equal to σ^2) against a uniform background in a slice or tomogram that would result from imaging annihilation events in positron emission tomography. Circular symmetry will be assumed and photon attenuation and detection inefficiencies (including MTF degradation) neglected. The uniform background level is written in the spatial domain as $f(x, y) = \overline{\rho}$, and the Gaussian lesion with peak amplitude $\Delta\rho$ is written as

$$\Delta f(x, y) = \Delta\rho \exp\left(-(x^2 + y^2)/2\sigma^2\right). \quad \text{(D.33)}$$

In the frequency domain this is just

$$\Delta\tilde{f}(\nu_x, \nu_y) = \Delta\rho \frac{a}{2} \exp\left(-(2\pi)^2(\nu_x^2 + \nu_y^2)\frac{\sigma^2}{2}\right) \quad \text{(D.34)}$$

where "a" represents the area $4\pi\sigma^2$

A projection of the lesion onto the x-axis in the spatial domain is equivalent to setting $\nu_y = 0$ in the Fourier domain, giving

$$\Delta\tilde{f}(\nu) = \Delta\rho\,\frac{a}{2}\exp\left(-(2\pi)^2\nu^2\sigma^2/2\right).\qquad\text{(D.35)}$$

This is a simple application of the projection-slice theorem given above. The subscript in Equation D.35 has been omitted since Δf may be taken as any radial component for the case of circular symmetry. If m views are taken and superimposed the spectrum becomes

$$\Delta\tilde{f}\to\Delta\tilde{f}\cdot\mathrm{F}_1(\nu).\qquad\text{(D.36)}$$

The SNR^2 for the ideal observer given the task of lesion detection specified above can now be calculated directly as

$$\mathrm{SNR}^2_{\mathrm{PET}} = \mathrm{C}^2\left\{\frac{a}{2}\right\}^2\frac{\bar{\rho}m}{Da^{1/2}},\qquad\text{(D.37)}$$

where $\mathrm{C} = \Delta\rho/\bar{\rho}$.

A similar expression would be obtained for x-ray CT if the analogy is made between the spatial density of the annihilation events and the spatial distribution of the attenuation coefficient. Notice that we have not required the use of a reconstruction algorithm to obtain this result. This would color the noise and the ideal observer would only undo this, essentially using the data in the original projections. The above result may also be obtained by using the filtered-back-projection algorithm to obtain the object and noise as imaged by such a procedure.

The previous example was one in which there was total uncertainty in the position of the annihilation event along the path of the line integral. Now consider the other limiting case for tomography, namely TOFPET imaging, in which the coincidence detection process has temporal resolution great enough to determine the position or range of the annihilation event. The SNR^2 per view is then simply

$$\mathrm{SNR}^2 = \mathrm{C}^2\left\{\frac{a}{2}\right\}^2\frac{\bar{\rho}}{a}\qquad\text{(D.38)}$$

and if the same total number of views, m, as used in the method of reconstruction from projections are

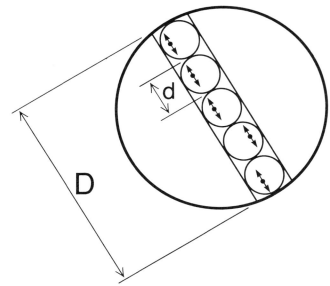

Fig. D.9. Origin of the multiplex penalty, with the noise from D/d lesion-size regions corrupting the strip integrals for each projection.

allowed, then one obtains the result

$$\mathrm{SNR}^2_{\mathrm{TOFPET}} = m\mathrm{C}^2\left\{\frac{a}{2}\right\}^2\frac{\bar{\rho}}{a}.\qquad\text{(D.39)}$$

If the ratio of Equation D.37 to Equation D.39 is taken, one finds

$$\mathrm{SNR}^2_{\mathrm{PET}}/\mathrm{SNR}^2_{\mathrm{TOFPET}} = a^{1/2}/D.\qquad\text{(D.40)}$$

In the limit of $a^{1/2}\to D$, a lesion the size of the format, this gives unity, or no gain from TOF information, which is obvious. In the other limit, $a\to 0$, the penalty for imaging *via* line integrals can be quite appreciable.

The inverse of the factor $a^{1/2}/D$ is the number of times the lesion can be laid across the object being imaged (see Figure D.9 where $d\approx a^{1/2}$). This is an effective noise multiplier — while signal is being collected from the lesion, noise is being collected from the entire strip integration. This factor is referred to as the linear noise-multiplex factor. This multiplexing, rather than any inefficiencies in the algorithm, is the reason for the high exposures required to carry out computed tomography.

WAGNER, R.F., INSANA, M.F., BROWN, D.G., GARRA, B.S. and JENNINGS, R.J. (1990a). "Texture discrimination: Radiologist, machine and man," page 310 in *Vision: Coding and Efficiency*, Blakemore, C., Ed. (Cambridge University Press, Cambridge, Massachusetts).

WAGNER, R.F., MYERS, K.J., BURGESS, A.E., BROWN, D.G. and TAPIOVAARA, K. (1990b). "Maximum a posteriori detection: Figures of merit for detection under uncertainty," *Proc. Soc. Photo-Opt. Instr. Eng.* **1232,** 195-204.

WATSON, A.B., BARLOW, H.B. and ROBSON, J.G. (1984). "What does the eye see best?" *Nature* **302,** 419-422.

WEAR, K.A., WAGNER, R.F. and GARRA, B.S. (1994). "High resolution ultrasonic backscatter coefficient estimation based on autoregressive spectral estimation," *IEEE Trans. Med. Imag.* (accepted for publication).

WEINSTEIN, M.C. and FINEBERG, H.V. (1980). *Clinical Decision Analysis* (Saunders, Philadelphia, Pennsylvania).

WHALEN, A.D. (1971). *Detection of Signals in Noise,* Electrical Science Series (Academic Press, New York).

WICKELGREN, W.A. (1968). "Unidimensional strength theory and component analysis of noise in absolute and comparative judgments," *J. Math. Psych.* **5,** 102-122.

WILCOX, G.W. (1968). *Inter-Observer Agreement and Models of Monaural Auditory Processing in Detection Tasks,* Ph.D. Dissertation (University of Michigan, Ann Arbor, Michigan).

WOLF, M. (1980). "Signal-to-noise ratio and the detection of detail in non-white noise," *Photog. Sci. and Engr.* **24,** 99-103.

WU, Y., DOI, K., METZ, C.E., ASADA, N. and GIGER, M.L. (1993). "Simulation studies of data classification by artificial neural networks: Potential applications in medical imaging and decision making," *J. Dig. Imag.* **6,** 117-125.

YAO, J. and BARRETT, H.H. (1992). "Predicting human performance by a channelized Hotelling observer model," *Proc. Soc. Photo-Opt. Instrum. Eng.* **1768,** 161-168.

ICRU Reports

ICRU Reports are distributed by the ICRU Publications' office. Information on prices and how to order may be obtained from:

ICRU Publications
7910 Woodmont Avenue, Suite 800
Bethesda, Maryland 20814
U.S.A.
Phone (301) 657-2652
FAX (301) 907-8768

Copies of the reports may also be purchased from the following:

Mrs. Brigitte Harder
Konrad-Adenauer-Straße 26
D-37075 Göttingen
Germany
Phone (0551) 22612

Kazuya Yamashita, Ph.D.
The Japanese Society of Radiological Technology
Nijyo Plaza, 88 Nakagyo-Ku,
Nakagyo-ku, Kyoto 604
Japan

Prof. André Wambersie
Unité de Radiobiologie et Radioprotection
UCL-Cliniques St. Luc
Avenue Hippocrate, 54.69
B-1200 Brussels, Belgium
Phone (02) 764.54.68

Japan Radioisotope Association
28-45, Honkomagome 2-chome
Bunkyoku Tokyo 113, Japan

Dr. Torgil Möller
Regionale Tumörregistret
  Lasarettet
S-22185 Lund
Sweden

The currently available ICRU Reports are listed below.

ICRU Report No.	*Title*
10b	*Physical Aspects of Irradiation* (1964)
10f	*Methods of Evaluating Radiological Equipment and Materials* (1963)
12	*Certification of Standardized Radioactive Sources* (1968)
13	*Neutron Fluence, Neutron Spectra and Kerma* (1969)
15	*Cameras for Image Intensifier Fluorography* (1969)
16	*Linear Energy Transfer* (1970)
17	*Radiation Dosimetry: X Rays Generated at Potentials of 5 to 150 kV* (1970)
18	*Specification of High Activity Gamma-Ray Sources* (1970)
20	*Radiation Protection Instrumentation and Its Application* (1971)
22	*Measurement of Low-Level Radioactivity* (1972)
23	*Measurement of Absorbed Dose in a Phantom Irradiated by a Single Beam of X or Gamma Rays* (1973)
24	*Determination of Absorbed Dose in a Patient Irradiated by Beams of X or Gamma Rays in Radiotherapy Procedures* (1976)

Binders for ICRU Reports are available. Each binder will accommodate from six to eight reports. The binders carry the identification, ''ICRU Reports'', and come with label holders which permit the user to attach labels showing the Reports contained in each binder.

The following bound sets of ICRU Reports are also available:

Volume I. ICRU Reports 10b, 10c, 10f
Volume II. ICRU Reports 12, 13, 14, 15, 16, 17, 18, 20
Volume III. ICRU Reports 22, 23, 24, 25, 26
Volume IV. ICRU Reports 27, 28, 30, 31, 32
Volume V. ICRU Reports 33, 34, 35, 36
Volume VI. ICRU Reports 37, 38, 39, 40, 41
Volume VII. ICRU Reports 42, 43, 44
Volume VIII. ICRU Reports 45, 46, 47
Volume IX. ICRU Reports 48, 49, 50, 51

(Titles of the individual Reports contained in each volume are given in the list of Reports set out above.)

The following ICRU Reports were superseded by subsequent Reports and are now out of print:

ICRU Report No.	Title and Reference*
1	*Discussion on International Units and Standards for X-ray work*, Br. J. Radiol. **23,** 64 (1927).
2	*International X-Ray Unit of Intensity*, Br. J. Radiol. (new series) **1,** 363 (1928).
3	*Report of Committee on Standardization of X-ray Measurements*, Radiology **22,** 289 (1934).
4	*Recommendations of the International Committee for Radiological Units*, Radiology **23,** 580 (1934).
5	*Recommendations of the International Committee for Radiological Units*, Radiology **29,** 634 (1937).
6	*Recommendations of the International Commission on Radiological Protection and of the International Commission on Radiological Units*, National Bureau of Standards Handbook 47 (U.S. Government Printing Office, Washington, D.C., 1951).
7	*Recommendations of the International Commission on Radiological Units*, Radiology **62,** 106 (1954).
8	*Report of the International Commission on Radiological Units and Measurements (ICRU) 1956*, National Bureau of Standards Handbook 62 (U.S. Government Printing Office, Washington, D.C., 1957).
9	*Report of the International Commission on Radiological Units and Measurements (ICRU) 1959*, National Bureau of Standards Handbook 78 (U.S. Government Printing Office, Washington, D.C., 1961).
10a	*Radiation Quantities and Units,* National Bureau of Standards Handbook 84 (U.S. Government Printing Office, Washington, D.C., 1962).
10c	*Radioactivity* (1963)
10d	*Clinical Dosimetry,* National Bureau of Standards Handbook 87 (U.S. Government Printing Office, Washington, D.C., 1968).
10e	*Radiobiological Dosimetry,* National Bureau of Standards Handbook 88 (U.S. Government Printing Office, Washington, D.C., 1963).
11	*Radiation Quantities and Units* (International Commission on Radiation Units and Measurements, Washington, D.C., 1968).

14   *Radiation Dosimetry: X Rays and Gamma Rays with Maximum Photon Energies Between 0.6 and 50 MeV* (1969)

19   *Radiation Quantities and Units* (International Commission on Radiation Units and Measurements, Washington, D.C., 1971).

19S   *Dose Equivalent* [Supplement to ICRU Report 19] (International Commission on Radiation Units and Measurements, Washington, D.C., 1973).

21   *Radiation Dosimetry: Electrons with Initial Energies Between 1 and 50 MeV* (International Commission on Radiation Units and Measurements, Washington, D.C., 1972).

29   *Dose Specification for Reporting External Beam Therapy with Photons and Electrons* (International Commission on Radiation Units and Measurements, Washington, D.C., 1978)

35   *Radiation Dosimetry: Electron Beams with Energies Between 1 and 50 MeV* (1984)

*References given are in English. Some of the Reports were also published in other languages.

Index